# HOW TO
# IMPROVE YOUR CHILD'S EYESIGHT NATURALLY

## A Thoughtful Parent's Guide

Janet Goodrich, Ph.D.

Healing Arts Press
Rochester, Vermont

Healing Arts Press
One Park Street
Rochester, Vermont 05767
www.InnerTraditions.com

Healing Arts Press is a division of Inner Traditions International

Originally published in Australia in 1996 by Sally Milner Publishing Pty Ltd., and in the United States in 1999
by Celestial Arts, under the title *Help Your Child to Perfect Eyesight Without Glasses*

*Note to the reader: This book is intended as an informational guide. The remedies, approaches, and techniques described herein
are meant to supplement, and not to be a substitute for, professional medical care or treatment. They should not be used to treat a
serious ailment without prior consultation with a qualified health care professional.*

**Library of Congress Cataloging-in-Publication Data**

Goodrich, Janet. (1942–1999)
  How to improve your child's eyesight naturally: a thoughtful parent's guide /
Janet Goodrich.
    p. cm.
  ISBN 0-89281-130-7
  1. Visual perception in children. 2. Low vision in
children—Patients—Rehabilitation.  I. Title.
  RE48.2.C5G667 2004
  617.7'0083—dc22

                            2003022302

Printed and bound in the United States at Capital City Press

10 9 8 7 6 5 4 3 2 1

Text design and layout by Rachel Goldenberg
This book was typeset in Janson Text with Triplex Serif as the display typeface

United Syndicate and Plenum Press kindly allowed reprint of copyrighted materials. All efforts have been made
to contact other original copyright holders. Any discrepancies will be altered upon notice. Thanks to the family
of Helen M. Kennedy for giving her Corbett materials to Janet Goodrich.

Illustrations: Veronica Davidson. Page 101, Fiona Whipp; pages 93 and 161, Chris Dent; page 179, Louise Coutts.
Photographs: page 70, S. Fredlyand; all other photos by Janet Goodrich or from her personal archives.
Technical consultants: The optometrists Adrian Bell, Bryan Smith, and Ross Fisher.
All songs and lyrics copyrighted ©1996 APRA, Austral-Asia Performing Rights Association. All rights reserved.

# Dear Reader,

Did your heart sink when you saw the report: "Your child's eyesight has been tested and found lacking. Please take him to an optometrist for an exam and glasses"? Do you still sigh and resign yourself to the sight of your bright-eyed child locked forever into a blurred world after a year or two in school? Does hearing that ever thicker glasses are normal and necessary make you grind your teeth?

Now you, a mere parent or grandparent, armed with only love and willingness, can turn a faulty vision report into a blazing adventure and miniature miracle for yourself and your child.

By taking one step at a time through this book, you and your whole family will gain a deeper understanding of the causes of blurred vision. Walking natural pathways to restoring clarity of eyesight will allow you to drop the crutches of optical devices along your way.

Rational explanations and insights are followed by a host of practical, easy vision-improvement games. Using and reusing this book will lighten your heart and get that child out of glasses!

Janet Goodrich

This book is for my beloved father,
Sidney Marcellus Goodrich

# Contents

# Part 3: Specific Programs for Specific Problems

## 13 Myopia

## 14 Hyperopia

# Acknowledgments

I wish to thank Cybele, Carina, and Aerro Goodrich-Harwell, my parents, childhood friends, and teachers. Children at Crystal Waters Permaculture Village and surrounding area grace these pages with their bright eyes. Local musicians Don Woodward, Bernard O'Scanaill, and Elizabeth Ledger gifted their music. Robin Harpley helped me with research. My husband, Geraldo, lent constant support on all fronts. Artists Veronica Davidson, Fiona Whipp, and Chris Dent brought words to life with images. I thank the optometrists and ophthalmologists who helped me with technical data. My heartfelt gratitude goes to Jill Morris, Amber, Dave, the Richardson family, Steve Wall and family, Elaine Wood, Grant Hammer, the children and parents at Playcamps, and especially the teacher trainees who relived their own childhood in the process of healing their sight.

My gratitude extends to the thousands of people who have had the courage and interest to receive, use, and pass on a greater truth about vision.

# Why I Wrote This Book

Ordinary citizens are longing to be directly active in preventing and reversing eyesight problems. Trained professionals are seeking a more human way of working with eyesight.

My suitcases were standing in the doorway, heavy with papers and books for the coming teacher training course in Germany. The phone rang. A woman in Newcastle described her nine-month-old grandson trying to crawl about the living room with glasses taped to his head and one eye covered with plaster. "It breaks my heart," she said. "Is there anything I can do to help him?"

Following my lecture in London at the Alternative Medicine Festival, a woman who does fusion training with children after strabismus operations grabbed my hand and moaned, "I have ten minutes with each baby. I really want to do something more with these children."

Upon arriving home I found a letter from Malaysia on my desk. An eight-year-old boy had just received his second pair of glasses within one year. His prescription had jumped from -5 to -8 diopters. Progressive myopia (nearsightedness) was the diagnosis, stronger glasses the only response. "Where will it end?" his mother wondered. In 1993 the government in Singapore spent thousands of dollars installing better lighting in classrooms, hoping somehow to hold back the tidal wave of myopia that sweeps 57 percent of all teenage boys in that country into glasses.

It is obvious that the automatic response of putting glasses on any child who manifests visual blur isn't helping. The possible causes of poor eyesight are ignored. Parents are left out of the picture altogether, except as check writers and enforcers of the "make her wear them all the time" rule. Most children's lifestyle, schooling, and diet are determined by mass marketing and cultural habits. Meanwhile you, as the producer and constant caregiver of the child, are written off as a dummy who should blindly obey the command: "Take the children for earlier and more frequent eye exams. But don't attempt any home remedies because you don't know enough."

The continuing frustration and apathy generated by the established optical industry challenged me and my myopic childhood. I had proudly sprouted glasses at age seven for myopia and astigmatism.

After twenty years behind coke-bottle-thick lenses, my inner being said, "Enough." Having used the Natural Vision Improvement processes myself, I discarded the glasses at age twenty-seven, passed all my vision tests without visual aids of any kind, and began to teach others to do the same. This child who shielded herself for twenty years behind a pair of glasses is tuning in to every child on this planet. She said "Write!" for the children who are going myopic, hyperopic, and cross-eyed. She said, "Tell parents children don't have to be put in glasses."

## Social and Optical Pressures

The dimming of once bright, sharp eyes is a signal to interact with your child. The artificial clarity of robot goggles obscures the constant opportunities to lead children toward naturally clear vision.

The pressure to use an optical solution is pervasive in our culture. Every day you will be confronted in your endeavor by voices and visuals denying the power to heal eyesight with natural means. Every shopping plaza sports an eyewear boutique. Schoolteachers have curriculum standards to maintain, tests to administer, and criticisms to beat. These good people are anxious to make sure the child performs well. Glasses, everyone knows, are required for adequate performance in the classroom. Grown-ups are relieved when the child can finally see and enjoy reading. Yet the signal flares are dulled. The glasses keep getting stronger. Cause is locked away in a back closet.

Be ready to deal with the disdain and patronizing righteousness of the optical experts. These folk are both well-meaning and trapped in their expensive training. Only licensed practitioners may diagnose the condition of the eye and determine the function of the visual apparatus of the human body. However, what you do with the diagnosis is up to you. You will probably hear, "There's nothing you can do to change this child's vision, except . . ." Interpret this as: "There is nothing I can do to change this child's vision except . . ." Do not let authoritarian opinions deter you. Imagine being a mouse eavesdropping on a conference open only to licensed doctors. You'd probably hear angry voices and the clash of one "scientific" belief system against another.

# A New Attitude

Many optometrists and even ophthalmologists have changed their minds about Natural Vision Improvement, using it themselves and recommending it to their patients.

I hold Janet Goodrich's book in my hand with delight and gratitude. It is an honor. A few years ago I would have rejected it out of hand. What I had learned in medical school was gospel. There are problems that can be healed and others that cannot. But the causes of the latter were all unknown, and I was not open to the possibility that "concrete facts" could be seen from another angle. Through my own experience I was led into another world, a new world of health and energy. On the nonphysical level powerful influences are active that orthodox medicine cannot reach. Often "incurable" illnesses disappear.

I wish from my heart that many people will use the playful and potent ideas in this book. Parents can sow many beneficial seeds for their children's vision while walking new and enjoyable pathways together.

*Editha Neumann, ophthalmologist, Germany*

We are living in times of great change. . . . Many people are increasingly dissatisfied with mechanical medicine and are deeply affected by the lack of time for explanation and human warmth from doctors. The great interest in alternative, gentler forms of therapy that speak to one's inner experience is growing accordingly.

The solution does not lie in "either-or." A valid answer comes only through a synthesis of both approaches. Janet Goodrich's book is a step in the right direction. Even established conservative eye doctors are beginning to see that the eye cannot be treated adequately when separated from mental and emotional considerations.

We ophthalmologists would do neither ourselves nor our patients a favor by rejecting the whole-person approach to vision in this book. The adage holds, "Whoever heals is right." Too often we assume that the previous measurements made by a colleague or optometrist were totally accurate. Every day in practice I encounter unexplainable changes in vision. Other areas of the body heal without mechanical intervention; why not eyesight?

I believe that this book, based on the author's many years of experience, offers everyone food for thought and valuable ways our patients can be helped, rather than prescribing yet another pair of glasses.

*Joy Patricia Wermann, ophthalmologist, Germany*

I am honored to write about this book. In the rising chorus of voices criti-cizing traditional ophthalmological and optometric treatment of functional vision problems, the voice of Janet Goodrich is worth listening to and has a clear message.

Consistent with well-documented vision research, Janet Goodrich pre-sents an elucidating educational progam. She speaks of the dynamic interplay between the child's eyes and the environment. In Janet's Method, mechani-cal devices—glasses and machinery—are used as little as possible. Her emphasis is on reconnecting the child (and the child within all of us) to the resources of life energy that are inherent in a joyful, exploring youth. These are the powerful resources that are obstructed during everyday life by the demands imposed on us all by education and society.

Our visual system is affected by every thought we think, the emotions we feel, and the movements we make. Twenty percent of the optic nerve fibers connect the light impulses coming from the eye to neural centers of atten-tion, emotion, body tone, movement, and posture. Our eyes are connected to every cell in our body! Janet Goodrich's vision-games method—encour-aging good vision through free movement, visualizations, emotional resolu-tion, and relaxation—is indeed related to excellent seeing.

Traditional ophthalmologists and optometrists reading this book will need the scientific data available from behavioral optometry to intellectually cross over to the promising land of Janet Goodrich's Natural Vision Improvement. For children and their parents, the entry into this land will be easy.

*Willemien Manschot, ophthalmologist, behavioral optometrist, the Netherlands*

# How to Use This Book

You have several ways to make this book a good friend and helpful guide:

- Read it from cover to cover.
- Use it as a referral book for subjects of interest, such as switching on the whole brain or finding out why the eye must move to see clearly.
- Activate the suggested game plans suited to your child's age and vision. All vision games and exercises are in bold headers with a graphic representation of an eye in the table of contents and text for quick reference.
- Sing. A child's first experience with music makes a permanent impression that can be called upon anytime in life for healing. The thirty-two songs in this book have the power to transmute the inhumanity that we all encounter. They are designed to saturate your lifestyle and make the games easier to use. You and your children can sing and hum these tunes silently or aloud anywhere, anytime: in the car, on holidays, strolling down the hallway at school.
- Plan, record, and share your experience.

Please read all the chapters in the book, even when they do not apply specifically to your child. Explanations given in one chapter will refine your understanding of an item touched upon somewhere else.

The timetables included in each activity chapter help you introduce a particular game at the right time in your child's development. Your child may be older than the suggested starting point. This does not mean that activity is irrelevant. For example, Holding Points starts at birth and continues through one's lifetime. The plus (+) sign after the month or year in the timetable means "carry this activity forward," regardless of age.

I use the word *you* throughout this book. The being to whom this "you" refers is variable. In explanatory text it refers to you yourself, as parent or teacher. In descriptions of vision games, it signifies the child or children listening as you read the section aloud.

# Who Can Benefit from Using This Book?

People with normal vision can use the activities in this book to increase their visual acuity. Future problems can be prevented by instilling good visual habits now.

Any child with blurred vision will benefit from using my Natural Vision Improvement program. Guidelines are given for parents and caregivers to reverse common refractive errors. If you are the adult leading the adventure to clear sight, consider following the program yourself. Sharing the experience is more effective than playing supervisor.

The vision-improvement games are meant to become part of your family lifestyle. All the relatives can join in. Grandparents take children to the park for Cross-Crawl dancing and Magic Pencil games. Mothers relax and revive themselves while holding reflex points on their babies. Brothers and sisters with normal vision love playing Pirate Patch with a cross-eyed sibling. Schoolteachers can calm themselves down with massage and yawning while children palm and visualize stories read to them. The possibilities for integrating the games contained in this book into daily life are endless.

# Guidelines to Keep in Mind

- Watch. Observe. Play with the little ones.
- Learn the vision-improvement games described in this book and apply them through the child's growing years.
- Enjoy a few minutes of quality time with your child each day while you both relax and play vision games together.
- Let go of the fear that your child won't be able to keep up in school or on the playground.
- Form a play group with friends and neighbors to do Janet's vision-improvement activities.
- Introduce Natural Vision Improvement to your sphere of acquaintances and practitioners.
- After one or two activities have become part of your family life, introduce some new games. Take your time. Enjoy the journey!

# How This Book Is Organized

## Part One: A Fresh View of Children's Vision

## (Chapters 1 to 5)

Here you will find the history of Janet's Method, theories of cause, and suggestions for dealing with optical professionals. Chapter 4 offers you a
blueprint for planning and record keeping in the innovative "Home
Science" project. Share your success. Only a few parents are audacious
enough to buck the system and consistently apply self-healing methods with
their children. Please let us know about the obstacles to your success and
how you overcome them.

The developmental stages of mental and visual growth are given in chapter 5, helping you to decide when to introduce specific vision activities. The
pace and comfort of the child is paramount at all times. Do not force or
frighten children into doing what you think they should do. Rather than saying, "If you don't do your vision games, your eyes will get worse and you'll
have to go back to glasses," you could say, "On Saturday let's go to the park
and do some Near-Far Swings on the swings.

Celebrate small victories. A half second of straight eyes or a flash of clarity deserves applause. One incredulous father said, "Maybe it's the change in
the light" when his myopic six-year-old daughter named all the animals on
the wall chart. She had not been able to identify them the day before. To me
this little girl's ability to see the animals clearly without glasses was a normal
miracle.

## Part Two: Keen Eyesight for Every Child

## (Chapters 6 to 12)

Learn the subtle power of reflex points and massage. Plunge into switching on
the brain with Cross-Crawl, then do Swings, Sunning, Palming, and other
vision games to foster good vision for yourself, your children, and everyone
else in your family or classroom. All the fundamental vision-improvement
games are explained and presented. These activities will enhance normal vision
and act as a preventive to future eyestrain. They are the basis for helping children out of glasses. This section also gives you a unique way to recognize and
help children with the emotions that are always tied to eyesight problems.

## Part Three: Specific Programs Specific Problems
## (Chapters 13 to 17)

Use part 3 to:

- Design a program for a child who has been diagnosed with abnormal vision by an optometrist or ophthalmologist.
- Find out more about the condition your child has manifested.
- Learn which activities are pertinent to your child. Begin slowly and easily with the suggested games, adapting them to your child's age and your personal daily routine. One vision game a month may be perfect.
- Experiment. First put the basic principles of good vision outlined in part 2 in your mind. Understand why, for example, movement is important for reversing myopia. Then you and your child can invent highly personal vision games.
- Record the information outlined on pages 33–34, keeping medical records and personal diary notations to document your progress with specific eye problems.

## Part Four: Home and School Environments
## (Chapters 18 to 20)

The design of diets, rooms, and learning and study spaces can be crucial to the development of good vision. Modern schooling is a most unnatural process. The child sits immobilized at a desk, often in front of a flat computer screen. Eyesight and happiness both suffer. Take ideas from part 4 to educators and teachers. Urge them to provide environments that build vision rather than destroy it.

At the end of this book is a resource section to help you go shopping for toys, tools, and materials to create a colorful and inspiring environment for your child. There is a section for recommended reading on related topics. You will also find information on seminars and instructor training. Referral addresses for Natural Vision Improvement (NVI) teachers and other helpful practitioners are available from NVI. You'll find the address at the back of this book.

## No More Glasses

The vision-improvement games are generally played without glasses or contact lenses. Eye charts, books, or drawing games can be placed as close or as far away as necessary for the child's ease of seeing.

If the child's vision needs optical help, weaker-than-normal Transition Glasses can be obtained. These T-Glasses allow the child to function like everyone else and still give the eyes room to change for the better. Even when using Transition Glasses for school or special situations, the vision games continue. The Magic Nose Pencil and Near-Far Swings are excellent for chalkboards and computers while using weaker corrective lenses. The guidelines for obtaining Transition Glasses are in chapter 3 (pages 23–25).

Part 1

# A Fresh View
# of Children's Vision

# 1

# People and Glasses

## A Brief History of Glasses

The prescribing and selling of glasses is a major world industry. Most of the people involved in this industry, and their customers, take it for granted that glasses are the best thing since sliced bread. If spectacles can be a fashion item, even better. Glasses, contact lenses, and a sixteen-second operation to shorten the myopic eyeball are helping millions of people compensate for their visual distress.

Alexander Da Spina, a monk living in the thirteenth century, may have put the first lenses into a frame. In the Middle Ages the wearing of glasses was a status symbol for the wealthy and intellectual segment of society. These polished stones were available from guilds and consisted of magnifiers enabling older people to read. Painters in the Renaissance depicted biblical figures wearing the latest Italian models.

Ever since ocular anesthesia was invented in 1884, it has been possible to place thin curved lenses onto the cornea at the front of the eye. Today plastic lenses float on a layer of tears in the eyes of more than 12 million Americans. However, extended-wear contact lenses have inherent problems. Bacteria build-up behind the lens can cause blinding infections. Corneal cells sometimes become oxygen starved and ulcerated. Newer contact lenses have tiny holes that oxygen molecules can penetrate.

Technologists produce better ocular aids all the time. However, I still recommend that Natural Vision Improvement students do not use contact lenses. Frames are more convenient to leave off and are harder to lose. Although contacts provide more peripheral vision, they deaden sensation and expressive feeling experienced through the eyes.

With glasses or contacts as the only answer, poor eyesight either stays the same or worsens. Without these optical crutches, human beings would have had to acknowledge and alter the stress factors that cause vision to degenerate in the first place.

# Children in Glasses

Before the industrial revolution and compulsory schooling, a booming market for children's glasses did not exist as it does today. Current statistics reveal an alarming rise in the number of children with vision problems.

The American Optometric Association Task Force on Optometric Manpower in 1990 published the following estimates:

In the age group 0–4, 10 percent have refractive problems (myopia, hyperopia, astigmatism). Seven percent of these preschoolers have binocular problems.

In the age group 5–16, this number rises to 18 percent for refractive error and 8 percent for binocular problems.

By the time these children are 17–24 years of age, the numbers rise to 39 percent.

*The Catholic Digest* (November 1980) reported that 40 percent of Americans wear glasses or contact lenses for myopia, in contrast to 18 percent of the population in 1939.

This number is increasing as "school myopia" becomes more prevalent. Hyperopia (farsightedness) and lack of eye coordination are also of concern. Children are spending less time manipulating manual toys and more time in front of computers. This causes loss of eye-hand coordination and disturbs the act of fusion during formative years. The optical industrialists call for infant eye exams; earlier detection of amblyopia ex anopsia, or "lazy eye"; and prompt treatment with glasses or eye-muscle surgery.

In this picture Janet is six years old. Her eyes are still soft and seeing clearly.

A twelve- to twenty-year school experience results in distorted bodies and dulled spirits. If the school is damaging the child, why not change the school and what happens in the classroom? The Optometric Association in Adelaide, Australia, is training teachers to detect vision disorders. These teachers could also be taught daily visual relaxation games. In Chinese factories and schools there is a pause each day to massage the acupuncture points related to eyesight.

Since the early 1920s, a few scientific and medical thinkers have protested the standard response of prescribing glasses when a child or adult demonstrated visual blur. Vehemently rejected or silently ignored, the work of these people has nonetheless been sought out by thousands of ordinary folks who feel there must be a better way to see.

# The Beginning of the Janet Goodrich Method

I was eager to go to school. Wonderful loving teachers in the small country schools I attended smiled at me through their glasses. I sat in the square desk assigned to me, contentedly playing with my scissors and crayons. But in the midst of this joy, anxiety about succeeding and being perfect was growing inside me. By the time I was seven, I could no longer read the blackboard. When the annual school photos were taken, I refused to wear my glasses. Eventually I looked like a stranger without them.

The bridge of my nose carries the memory of metal-framed glasses. Perhaps my mother trusted none of the available optical professionals; she took me to a different one each year. The optometrists praised me for being polite, quiet, and obedient. They told my mother I had an interesting pair of eyes and that the previous optometrist had given me the wrong prescription. I was soon unable to read, play ball, or get the dishes clean without my specs. My eyes became slits. I refused to look at my school photos.

At age eleven Janet was described as a "shy and sober but highly intelligent child."

At thirteen I had to leave the country school where I had been the only child in my grade for seven years. I could no longer do a semester of schoolwork within the first month and spend the remaining time reading and building hay nests in the school yard. Playing teacher to the little kids was over. High school closed in around me like a straitjacket. I was too visible. I survived the internal pressure with academic achievement. Less than an A on a report card meant burning at the stake. Darell Boyd Harmon had described me perfectly in his observations of American schoolchildren. I had all of his typical symptoms: digestive problems ("All little girls have stomachaches," the village M.D. told my worried mother); aching, scratchy eyeballs behind my specs; frequent colds and pneumonia.

University was the only alternative for farm girls with high IQs. Either that or get married—or get a job with General Motors and then get married. My mind was working overtime. I decided I would never cry. By age twenty-one I was using -7 diopters in front of my right eye and -5 diopters in front of the left for nearsightedness and astigmatism. One eye pulled up and the other down. At the University of Michigan hospital an ophthalmologist refused to give me contact lenses. He said my right cornea was too distorted with astigmatism. Using contacts could result in scarring. I wanted to do gymnastics and kung fu. The heavy frames slid down my face. A street-corner optometrist in Los Angeles was happy to sell me a pair of contacts. The physical pain as I tried to get used to the contacts is etched in my mind. I lost them within three days. The pain was telling me something. I didn't know what the message was. I'd been told, "Once a myope, always a myope."

In this picture the blur-producing stare is well in place and the smile is frozen. The glasses guard the eyes and brain from perceiving too much.

## Those Who Wanted Children out of Glasses

Two major teachers appeared in my life. Both these men had died before I was old enough to seek them out in person. I followed the spoor of their lives' work. The first major influence was the psychiatrist and biological scientist Wilhelm Reich (1897–1957). Reich had been declared a "medical charlatan" by a U.S. federal judge in 1955. Doctor Reich was a student of Sigmund Freud. He parted company with that august figure, deciding that people are more afraid of pleasure than of death. Reich's ideas were violently rejected by the medical and political fraternity of his era. His ideas took seed, in spite of the burning of his inventions and publications by the U.S. government in 1956.

Reich's ideas about child raising are found everywhere today: natural childbirth, breast-feeding babies, giving teenagers their own rooms, open and natural sexuality, the deliberate encouragement of self-regulation and aliveness in children. Reich lived and died for these ideals.

"If I am put in jail I will die," he stated. The judge who sentenced Reich to two years for contempt of court declared Reich's lifework in biology and psychiatry fraudulent—because "life energy does not exist."

Suppression of natural human feelings will result in chronic muscular tension in the body. There are six large muscles outside and two smaller intricate muscles inside the eye. All perception of life is distorted by this muscular "armoring." In his writings, Reich described how human beings would relate to one another if they were not shielded by chronic muscular and emotional patterns:

> They would identify with one another on the basis of the sensations of movement and rhythm. Contempt for natural movements would be foreign to them, just as they would have no comprehension of unnatural behavior. Development would be provided for and guaranteed through the continuous production of internal energy, as in the budding of flowers. . . . Moreover, there would be no end to the development. *Achievement would be within the framework of general biological activity; it would not be at variance with it.* [emphasis mine]

Wilhelm Reich,
psychiatrist

A smog-spewing Ford carried me to Los Angeles seeking a therapy for the body rather than for my top-heavy intellect. I wanted to be free of myopia and the constant sensation that I was not really alive. My Reichian therapist in Los Angeles took one look at my squinty eyes and said, "Start breathing—and get rid of your glasses." I blinked and sobbed without knowing why. Philip Curcuruto, D.C., fostered my breathing and the melting of my body armor. I had to find a way to get rid of my glasses myself. I sought out the work of American ophthalmologist William H. Bates (1860–1931). Dr. Bates published a book called *Perfect Eyesight without Glasses*. With his wife, Emily Lierman, Bates helped hundreds of children to better vision without glasses in their New York City clinic.

In the 1940s the Bates Method was made illegal in the state of New York. Although Bates's ideas are still predictably spat upon by those who sell glasses, a revised edition of his book sells steadily around the world. In the modern reprints the original copyright date of 1920 has been removed.

I have *Better Eyesight* magazines by Bates, and his wife's book *Stories from the Clinic*. These publications are packed with anecdotes of children improving their sight with a few visual imagery and relaxation activities. The following is an excerpt from Emily Lierman's book. (Please note that she frequently uses the word *cure*. Nowadays the word *cure* is a no-no for anyone who is not a licensed medical practitioner.)

> Then a mother came to the clinic with her two little girls. Marjorie, the older, had been to us some years previously and was cured. . . . The mother

kept looking at me, smiling all the while. She asked: "Don't you remember me? Don't you remember my little girl? I brought her to you and Dr Bates six years ago. She had alternate squint when she was three years old, and Dr Bates cured her without an operation." . . . Her sister Katherine, age seven years, stood by, wondering what we were going to do with her. Dr Bates examined her and said she had myopia, but not a bad case.

I placed her ten feet from the test card and she read every letter correctly down to the 20/40 line. As I walked over to where the card was placed to assist my little patient, the mother went ahead of me and in a soft tone of voice encouraged Katherine to palm and remember the last letter of the 20/40 line of the card. Katherine did so, but she had only covered her eye for a minute when she removed her hands and opened her eyes to read again. I wanted to tell the child that she had not palmed long enough, but before I could say a word, she began to read the next line of letters as her mother pointed to each one. After each letter was read, her mother very gently told her to blink and that would help her to see the next letter without a strain.

When Katherine had finished reading all of the 20/30 line without a mistake, the mother did not stop, but kept right on to the next line, pointing to one letter and then another until she read all of the 20/20 line. Then the mother advised Katherine to swing her body from side to side and to notice that everything in the room seemed to move in the opposite direction. While her mother was advising her what to do, the child did the best she could to read the card. The mother smiled when she saw how amazed I was to see her improve Katherine's eyes without my help. I asked: "Where did you learn how to do it?" She answered: "From reading your articles in the 'Better Eyesight Magazine.' I have been a subscriber for a number of years."

Some months later I saw them again. Katherine's vision was 20/20 in each eye. It is interesting to report that the child was cured entirely by her mother.

William H. Bates,
ophthalmologist

I found remnants of the Bates Method in the Los Angeles suburbs. After her husband had been saved from blindness using Bates's techniques, Margaret Corbett (1890–1960) established the School of Eye Education in Los Angeles. Four vision teachers trained by Margaret Corbett were still active in LA when I arrived on the scene. One of these teachers peered at her callers from behind a locked door. She was afraid of arrest. Margaret Corbett had been tried twice for practicing optometry without a license. Aldous Huxley, author of a lovely book on the Bates Method called *The Art of Seeing*, had testified at Corbett's trial. The charges against Mrs. Corbett were

Margaret Darst Corbett

dropped both times. State legislators refused to pass a bill prohibiting the teaching of the method. Nonetheless, fresh investigations could happen at any moment. Board of Optometry officials and busybodies who didn't want to think vision training could exist outside a few optical devices continued to harass and condemn lay practitioners of the Bates Method.

I was grateful for sessions with Hilda Reach, who had been the youngest in her Corbett training class. She revealed that Corbett teachers, who had once numbered fifty in Los Angeles alone, had disbanded their association in 1960 on the advice of a lawyer.

During the fifteen years I taught my version of the Corbett-Bates method in Los Angeles, I worked with several thousand people through classes and lectures. A jittery Chicano woman came to me for a private vision session. She turned out to be an undercover agent for a government bureau. Who is this person daring to talk about eyesight without an O.D. after her name?

I was driving daily on the Los Angeles freeway system. I needed the help of optometrists to weaken my glasses. The fellow who assisted me did so under duress. Within two years I was able to pass my California driving test without glasses. I have been free of frames and glasses ever since. I also take exception to the use of bifocals for people over forty. I don't need correction for reading.

My life has been devoted to helping adults and children out of glasses. I regularly train people from all walks of life to do the same. There is no faculty for this at any college, although one certified teacher is giving Natural Vision Improvement classes at Monash University. The belief system that says "There's no solution except glasses" has to be circumvented on a personal level.

My doctoral thesis in psychology dealt with visual armoring. It became clear to me that when Bates wrote of relaxation of the mind, he was talking about emotions. Mental stress is emotional stress. Reich's insights made it obvious that myopia in particular has a feeling component. I joined in the formation of a school that fostered expression of feelings and self-regulated learning. My children attended this school while I was teaching vision-improvement classes and training as a Reichian therapist.

## Honored Voices Ignored

I visited the biomedical library at UCLA with a forged pass. The books of Arnold Gesell, M.D., Darell Boyd Harmon, Alfred Yarbus (a Russian researcher in eye movements), and Sir Stewart Duke-Elder (ophthalmologist to Queen Elizabeth II) fell into my hands. These men are all highly honored names in the fields of optometry and medical science. I was greatly puzzled. Their recommendations are not put into practice.

The holistic conclusions of Gesell, Harmon, and Duke-Elder did not make it through the standardized and licensed "refract and prescribe" habit of the optical industry. Reading the original writings of the above-mentioned gentlemen is inspiring. Arnold Gesell, pediatric ophthalmologist, observed the visual behavior and development of fifty children from birth to age ten at the Yale Clinic of Child Development. He writes:

> Human visual perception ranks with speech in complexity and passes through comparable developmental phases. Moreover, seeing is not a separate, isolated function: it is profoundly integrated with the total action system of the child: posture, manual skills and coordination, intelligence and even personality make-up. Indeed, vision is so intimately identified with the whole child that we cannot understand its economy and hygiene without investigating the whole child.

In 1938 the Texas State Department of Health started a long-range survey of children in classrooms. An inventory was made of 160,000 elementary-school children; physical aspects of more than four thousand classrooms were noted. Darell Boyd Harmon published the results: "Analysis of the data showed that at least 52 per cent of the elementary school children were leaving the school with an average of 1.8 observable preventable defects per child." We will visit classrooms again in chapter 20.

Alfred Yarbus researched saccadic eye movements. At the end of his book *Eye Movements and Vision* he states, "People who think differently also, to some extent, see differently." The philosophical conclusions of Doctors Gesell, Harmon, Yarbus, and Reich colored the evolution of the Janet Goodrich Method. The ideas of these gentlemen are sprinkled throughout this book; they mingle congenially with the lifelong works of Reich, Bates, Emily Lierman-Bates, and Margaret Corbett.

The techniques of John Thie, D.C., founder of Touch for Health and author of a book by the same name, entered the picture. An evolving understanding of meridians, reflex points, and the balancing of mind and body energy seeped into NVI. Some of educator Paul Dennison's work with dyslexic children was added to the program.

While driving alone one day on the busiest freeway in the world, I heard a voice loud and clear: "You must once again live where everything is green." Responding to an invitation to live and teach in Australia, I loaded my three children onto an airplane.

During this time I wrote the book *Natural Vision Improvement*. This was first published in Australia and is now available in the United States, Germany, France, Spain, and Slovakia.

Eventually the emerald green landing pad of my dreams in California appeared, nestled in the hinterland of Queensland's Sunshine Coast. Crystal Waters is a Permaculture housing development devoted to care of people and care of the earth. Forty-five children live in this valley community: none of them need glasses. They attend vision play sessions for knowledge and entertainment. The Natural Vision Improvement Center now stands here, surrounded by thousands of young trees.

## A Natural Way to Healing

The child heals innocently. Children lie down with a fever, do not eat for a day or so—and recover their balance. Love, support, and knowledge will help keep adults from interfering with this natural process. Self-love will keep us looking for causes behind symptoms and ways to support the healthy growth of the child rather than accept the anesthesia of glasses. Dr. Duke-Elder wrote in his book *The Practice of Refraction:*

> Nothing is more pernicious than the routine correction of optical defects by rule-of-thumb methods. The matter is much more subtle and far-reaching. Many symptoms which are apparently caused by refractive errors or muscular anomalies would give no trouble in the ordinary course of events. They become apparent only because of ill-health or because of doing more work than the individual is capable of accomplishing with ease. A frequent instance of this is the troubles of which many children complain when commencing the routine of school life. If a rest and general tonic treatment are prescribed, these symptoms frequently disappear without any help in the form of glasses.
>
> . . . If the latter alone are prescribed and the warning of overwork as manifested in the eyes is neglected, the glasses may provide the patient with the means whereby to struggle on until he suffers a much more serious breakdown. The adjustment of suitable lenses is not sufficient treatment in itself.

# 2

# Causes of Imperfect Eyesight

## What Is Eyesight?

Definitions determine actions. If seeing is a mechanical function, then a trip to the optical shop for a new pair of lenses will be satisfactory.

Honoring eyesight as a living, changing expression intimately reflecting the child's inner life will change your tactics when visual blur appears. You will hunt for the source of the problem. Glasses are given as a response to symptoms. Automatically popping glasses on children allows everyone to ignore the cause and disdain a real solution.

A retinoscope

## Who Says It's Faulty?

Optical practitioners prescribe glasses using two different kinds of assessment. The first is a subjective test. The child must identify letters or shapes printed in black and white on a flat card. The second part of the examination is retinoscopy, which detects refractive error in the eyeball.

The retinoscope reflects light bouncing off the retina of the eye in such a way that the practitioner can tell you if an eye is too long, as in myopia, or too short, as in hyperopia. A competent practitioner will combine these subjective and objective methods to produce an adequate prescription.

This eyeball is too long = myopia.

This eyeball is "normal."

## Testing Vision Creates Blur

Does the test process itself create stress and visual blur? Reading an eye chart demands left-brain performance. Being peered at with an instrument is threatening to most children. When only the left brain is called into play, the

This eyeball is too short = hyperopia.

visual system contracts. Fear of failure and stage fright will affect the result. Through his retinoscope Dr. Bates saw a child's normal eyes turn myopic. Swinging around, he glimpsed a boy from the neighborhood staring at his patient through the window.

The attitude and manner of the person doing the testing can also affect the results. A patient handed his previous prescription to Ken Chenery, O.D. It was far stronger than the refractive error that Ken had just found in the man's eyes. Ken asked what had happened during the examination. "The optometrist was in a hurry," was the response. Ken concluded, "Sometimes people produce myopia to please optometrists."

A child trying to read black-and-white letters or numerals is under acute pressure to give the right answers. Susan Baker at age eight resisted the test itself. "My vision is good," she asserted to the school nurse. She was forced to read the chart. Her mother bought a pair of glasses. Susan threw her specs into the ditch. One year later an optometrist found she had completely normal vision.

Many visual faculties are not part of the normal vision test. Color, depth, and contrast perception are not addressed. Optical measuring cannot judge the aliveness, the sparkle, of the child's visual actions. To many doctors, personal and parental observation is "not scientific" and doesn't count. However, only a lightly armored adult will see aliveness in a child and remark upon its presence.

## Vision Fluctuates

Visual perception changes from moment to moment. I am baffled that optical professionals ignore this fact. People with normal eyesight frequently notice that fatigue, illness, or an argument will blur their vision temporarily.

Within the space of one month, attorney John Rock took his five-year-old son, Cheney, to three different ophthalmologists. All of them reported that Cheney was extremely hyperopic and needed to wear glasses all the time. Their prescriptions for Cheney varied from +2 to +5 diopters of correction. Cheney's dad did not buy glasses. He elected to take time from his hectic LA law practice to play vision-improvement games on the beach with his son. Six months later, a fourth ophthalmologist examined Cheney's eyes. There was no refractive error to be found.

# Theories Proposed and Rejected

The cause of hyperopia and astigmatism is rarely discussed in professional literature. Only recently have lack of eye coordination and reading stress been linked to computer use.

Theories about myopia abound, however, and there is little agreement about what produces it. If your practitioner has a pet theory, please realize there are other prestigious and opposing opinions.

## Myopia Is Inherited

Two kinds of studies deny the inheritance theory: first, surveys show that identical twins are not both myopic. Second, the eyes of Canadian Eskimos were examined over three generations. Only 5 percent of the eldest generation displayed distance blur, whereas 65 percent of their grandchildren were showing elongated eyeballs. The Eskimo research gave support to the "conditions of use" theory of myopia because the grandchildren were put into missionary schools to get a proper British education.

## Myopia Is Caused by "Conditions of Use"

"Reading for too long at an early age produces a spasm in the accommodative muscle of the eye—the ciliary muscle. This chronic tension elongates the eyeball." Optometrists who adhere to this theory think that putting minus lenses on myopic children will result in more myopia. They would rather put these children in plus magnifying lenses, and in some cases bifocals, to relax the ciliary muscle. Another proposal was to make avid young readers do something else.

In the 1930s the "conditions of use" theory rationalized putting brilliant myopic youngsters at pottery wheels. Charles Kelley, founder of the Radix Institute in America, was a budding scientist who resented making clay pots when he wanted to read math books. Coercing this child into another occupation did not reverse his progressing myopia. With 20/400 vision at the end of high school, he became a teacher of the Bates Method. He discarded his glasses while attending university and paid for his education by teaching others to do the same. No one had asked him if he wanted the pots instead of the books.

## Don't Discuss Feelings

The Eskimo studies did not address emotional conditions. In North America indigenous children were separated from their parents and siblings, forced to speak only English, forbidden their native culture. The scientists who studied them were children of their own culture and unwilling to break its taboos. Wilhelm Reich worked long and hard to show that emotions, or life energy, moving through the organism will affect perception. When life energy is suppressed, the "ocular segment" is frozen and perception through the eyes deadened and distorted. Post-Reichian psychologists behind thick lenses writing their Ph.D.s on myopia felt free to ask if myopes share common emotional and personality characteristics.

Sure enough, they discovered that a lot of myopes read under the blankets at night. Myopes are teacher's pets and high academic achievers. They hate to make mistakes. Nearsighted children inhibit their impulses and hide their fear. They seldom risk their humor. In contrast, hyperopes throw wonderful temper tantrums. The young myope will think twice and convert her distress into a lengthy analysis.

One optometric researcher did draw a line between mental stress in school and myopia. Dr. G. W. Van Alphen suggested that the pressure of doing schoolwork starts in the higher centers of the mind-body structure. The brain shoots its "burn-out!" message through the autonomic nerve system. The right-brain relaxation response remains turned off. This reflex normally releases stressed mechanical structures inside the eye. Therefore it is very possible that when little kids suffer over their homework, the normalizing mechanism for the eyes is bypassed. This can result in chronic hyperopia and myopia.

## The World at Large

Any change in eyesight affects the way the child feels about herself and her place in the world. The cultural factors that come to bear on a child's eyesight are of prime importance. Social ethics, comments by adults, leisure outlets, and media messages all influence the child's values and choices.

An entrancing net is woven about the child in the home and on the streets. Blurred eyesight is presented both as stigma and as a sign of high IQ. The messages coming to the child are confused. Why, if the blond princess with perfect eyesight wins the prince, should I have to wear glasses? Why, if Superman is goofy in his specs and flies through the skies hero-fashion without them, must I carry clumsy devices on my face all the time?

Americans fear three things: death, public speaking, and blindness. Lack of physical vision brings no position of honor. "Put on your glasses or you will go blind" is an excellent way to manifest what is feared. The rush to find a cure or a compensation for poor vision is understandable.

Notice how wearing glasses can be subtly rewarded. At age seven Margaret Schultz pretended to be myopic. She deliberately misread the eye chart. Her older sister was good in school and wore glasses. "Dad loves her more. Now he will love me too." Margaret fell into her own trap. Her eyes produced myopia to accommodate the glasses. Taking her glasses off in an NVI seminar brought back this memory of her cause.

## The Real Cause of Faulty Vision

All of my experience and study tells me that visual blur is related to numerous intertwining factors.

Children lacking in self-love, for whatever reason, will seek approval from others. They contract their bodies and minds into tight knots to ensure faultless academic and social performance. Such children win the top prizes in class—and the myopic glasses.

I wish to bring the hush-hush issues of emotion, life energy, and self-expression back into the picture. Working with emotional factors even mildly has helped Natural Vision Improvement students resolve life issues that have haunted them since early childhood. Dealing with feelings changes myopic and hyperopic personality patterns. Children and their companion adults can be helped tremendously with simple Emotional Healing games, such as those given in chapter 11, that attend to their inner life.

Nutrition plays a part. Proteins, vitamins, and minerals compose the structure of living eyeballs. If an essential nutrient is missing or toxic substances are entering the body, developing vision can be affected. The brain, processing input from the eyes and other senses, needs proper nutrition and plenty of oxygen. Myopes tend to consume a lot of meat and sugar. White sugar affects the body's use of chromium, important to muscular function. In chapter 18 we will tackle the sugar challenge.

It is not normal for a child to have visual blur of any kind. *The child's environment, internal and external, causes poor vision.* Let us change that environment to the extent we are able. In chapter 5 you will have a preview of developing motor and visual skills. You will be able to enter the magical, wondrous world of the child with playful vision games that fit right into the life you enjoy together.

# 3

# The Optical Industry and Natural Vision Improvement

## Professional Offerings

The development of the optical industry has created three main classes of professionals: ophthalmologists, optometrists, and opticians. There is a fourth small group called orthoptists, who work under the supervision of ophthalmologists. It is important to distinguish among these groups and to know what each has to offer. The training and belief systems of the human beings working in these professions will affect the way your child's vision develops and the future of his eyes and mind.

The rules governing the practice of vision care vary with the country. In the United States and Australia one finds ophthalmologists and optometrists. Optometry does not exist in Germany but may do so in the future as the Common Market countries sort out the battle between already entrenched interest groups and the marketplace demands of their inhabitants. Orthoptics as a profession does not exist in many countries. Consulting the nearest library may help you to discover what services are available in your locality.

## Ophthalmologists Are Medical Doctors

Ophthalmology is a specialty branch within orthodox medicine. These medical doctors diagnose and prescribe drugs or surgery for eye diseases. They also measure eyesight for refractive errors and prescribe glasses. Opticians educated in the precision grinding of lenses fill the prescriptions. Orthoptists, predominantly women, offer children a course of eye exercises for fusion after surgery or as an adjunct to glasses.

The education of ophthalmologists is long and rigorous. In Australia students take a university degree in medicine lasting six years, followed by three years of internship. Those wishing to specialize in eyes join the Registrars of Ophthalmology, a four-year course with two sets of exams. There are 768 ophthalmologists with open practices in Australia. The American Academy of Ophthalmologists lists 20,000 members, with 570 of these working in pediatrics. These people are medical doctors.

"The ophthalmologist looked me straight in the eye and said, 'There is absolutely nothing else you can do for your boy's eye except surgery.' I didn't believe him," the young mother explained to me on the phone. "Simon only has a slight turn in one eye and when he is tired it gets worse. When he is happy and lively I can hardly notice the turn at all. So something must be changing." I referred this mother to a behavioral optometrist for another opinion as she started the Natural Vision Improvement program.

In Germany NVI teachers have taught people how to relax their eyes and improve vision in adult education schools. Annoyed by this for ten years, the ophthalmologists in that country issued an official paper titled "Myopia Cannot Be Trained Away."

In other countries the response of medical practitioners to the Bates Method and anything similar varies from outright horror, through ignorance of the method, to complete acceptance.

Probably most ophthalmologists will say, "It can't hurt you and it can't help you. But I will be happy to monitor your progress—if you make any."

At the other end of the rejection/acceptance spectrum stand a few medical doctors who are friends of Natural Vision Improvement. These unorthodox doctors give out eye exercises to their patients or recommend my method. They discuss nutrition with their patients. Some practice acupuncture. These rare doctors' names and addresses can be obtained from the NVI head office in Australia.

## Optometrists Are Everywhere

Qualifying as an optometrist in Australia requires completion of a four-year degree course at an approved university, followed by board registration. Optometrists are trained to recognize eye diseases and refer any disease cases to ophthalmologists. In the United States optometrists first complete a basic science degree, followed by four years of optometry school. These graduates set up a practice: you have seen their shop windows selling glasses. These folks carry O.D. after their names. In Asia optometrists/opticians learn the trade through apprenticeship with their relatives. They do not have formal university training; however, a college of optometry has now been set up in Malaysia with twenty-four students.

Approximately 28,000 people practice optometry in the United States. There are currently 2,345 optometrists in Australia.

Within the group of "straight" optometrists, there are "behavioral," or "developmental," optometrists. In Los Angeles an optometrist checking out my vision classes informed me that behavioral optometry was a "dying cult."

There are 250 very alive members of this "dying cult" in the country of Australia; between ten and twenty of them run clinics where your child can have vision training. The College of Optometrists in Vision Development in the United States lists 1,600 members, and there may be as many as 5,000 optometrists in that country who take a performance-based look at their patients' visual systems. Behavioral optometrists are usually willing to weaken glasses for NVI students and to keep track of their progress.

In the *Journal of Behavioral Optometry*, an article appeared entitled "Seeing Space—Undergoing Brain Re-programming to Reduce Myopia." Author Antonia Orfield, O.D., described reducing her myopic glasses over a period of seven years using a variety of lifestyle improvements such as nutrition, exercise, postural training, and chiropractic. Within the article is also a strong hint that putting myopic children into glasses may be counterproductive.

Seek out these optometrists to obtain weakened glasses and minimal support for your Natural Vision Improvement program. Do not expect them to agree totally with life energy concepts and leaving off glasses to allow visual and emotional change. These people like to make the changes happen with optical devices. From an information pamphlet: "Vision therapy serves to help patients strengthen the link between vision and intelligence. Through the use of lenses and activities, it provides a patient with both development and learning experiences. The patient experiences conditions in which the old inefficient visual habits are changed into new behaviors."

One notable exception to optometrists churning out lenses is Jacob Liberman, O.D., who no longer puts people in glasses at all. He dares to ask his fellow optometrists to take off their glasses and contact lenses in his seminars, measuring their vision improvement after twenty-four hours. The results are described in his book *Take Off Your Glasses and See*.

Even though mainstream optometry has steadily denied or ignored the work of lay practitioners of vision improvement from the 1920s to the present, they still could not deny that the students of these teachers could read the smallest letters on the charts without glasses. The response was standardized. The oft-repeated phrases were and still are: "You're just reinterpreting the blur. There is no real physical change." "You were measured incorrectly." Or, to the over-forties: "Your eyes just happen to be physiologically young."

The hostility of medical doctors and optometrists to Natural Vision Improvement and the Bates Method is based on disbelief in the usefulness of vision training and on the false assumption that Bates Method students are routinely encouraged to shun visits to eye doctors when they have diseases such as glaucoma. Only the foolish would ignore a disease condition, and vision training is now becoming more popular within the optical industry itself. The American Optometric Association claims that 44 percent of their twenty-five thousand members provide some form of visual training.

It would of course be possible for NVI teachers, ophthalmologists, and optometrists to work in harmony. Politics of several stripes intervene. An NVI student in Los Angeles, a dance therapist with high myopia, demonstrated great success with the program to her ophthalmologist. The doctor then wanted to refer other patients to me, but only in secret. Disbelief in natural methods, fear of malpractice charges, and peer pressure cause medical doctors to behave in their own fashion.

Times are changing. Six optometrists have taken the two-month Certified Instructor Training course in the Natural Vision Improvement Method, and some of these are conducting NVI classes for their patients.

## Natural Vision Improvement Method Teachers

Certified teachers who train with me are ordinary citizens who take a 240-hour instructors course plus practice teaching. This course includes anatomy and physiology, relaxation techniques for different kinds of functional visual blur, and techniques for avoiding the wrath of medical practitioners by not claiming to have a "cure" for anything. I insist that anyone with an eye disease seek out and remain under the care of a medical specialist. The emphasis in my method is on healing vision in a relaxed, knowledgeable, and practical fashion. Teacher trainees are exposed to the psychological factors and emotional-healing techniques that underpin visual styles and types. There is an ever-growing demand for NVI instructors around the world.

Hilary Graham, certified Natural Vision Improvement teacher in Adelaide, South Australia:

I usually take children from the age of six years onwards, and most of them have turned or just lazy eyes. I have had great success with these children. I think that children's eye muscles are more supple and respond very quickly, round about the fifth lesson. They also love doing their vision games. One little eight-year-old girl was practically blind in one eye. She didn't wear glasses, as the eye specialist said that the eye was too far gone. On her fourth lesson she could read the bottom line on the close card with a patch on her good eye. Her distant vision also improved with that eye.

# How to Help Your Eye Doctor Give You What You Want

The flaming issue for you is how to obtain support for doing a home vision program from whichever optical professional you visit. Eye exams are needed for diagnosis and objective documentation. I personally prefer the idea of using optical devices as little as possible, but weaker lenses are often needed while eyesight is improving. The alternative to using glasses when some kind of visual aid is needed is to purchase pin-hole spectacles. Pin-hole spectacles are not prescription items, as they do not bend light. They are available in some health food stores and by mail order from us.

The parent groups at our Vision Playcamps have brought up two themes that keep them from dealing confidently with the optical professionals. The first factor is childhood training. When you step into a clinic do you hear your mother's voice saying, "Be quiet, don't bother the busy man" or your dad's voice: "Stop asking so many questions"?

The second factor is that both optometry and ophthalmology are exclusive clubs that inherited the Sophist style of schooling. To create such a school you first build a wall, put a sign outside the single door, and make people pay a high entry fee to enter. Once you've paid your money, memorized texts through long dark nights, and sweated blood to serve humanity, you reenter the "real" world to open a clinic. Ninety-nine percent of the humans who have been through the mill to get a degree are unwilling to question the validity of what they learned in the process.

The desire on your part to blank out and say, "He must know what he is doing," can keep you from winning an ally inside the club. This could make a big difference in your child's vision. As a parent you have every right to question your professional friend, receiving plain English answers until you have complete understanding of your child's situation. Blanking out and not asking the questions that haunt you in the middle of the night also allows you to lay blame on the doctor who "should have known better." Blaming others is the space-age way of throwing options down the toilet. And don't be bamboozled by the phrase "It's not scientific."

The denial of the value of your own experience is made official in the statement "There's no scientific proof" . . . that vision-improvement activities will improve vision problems. People who have experienced a "flash" of clear vision without glasses, while doing one of the games in this book, know that trying to prove to a skeptic that they are seeing with crystal clarity is the surest way to fall back into the blur.

## The Office Visit

Tell the receptionist when you make the appointment that you intend to do home vision training with your child. She can then allot extra time for your visit. Certain days and times are slower than others in the clinic. Pick a slow time to ask all your questions.

Tell the receptionist that you will be coming to interview the doctor. It is your right. Take paper and pen with you plus the following questions. The answers to these questions will form part of your Home Science records. Ask about vision in general and your child's vision in particular.

When you make the appointment use the following checklist:

- How long will my child be with the doctor? (Richard Kavner, O.D., in his book *Your Child's Vision*, states that a complete vision exam for a child should take between forty-five minutes and two hours.)
- Find out if the practitioner is interested in any background on the child: your pregnancy, the birth, the medical history of child and parents. These are important factors in the visual history of your child.
- Ask exactly what kinds of visual abilities the child will be tested for.
- What are the doctor's goals in treating children's vision?

- Ask for a written report in plain English, rather than scrawled medicalese. Make sure you obtain a copy of any prescription and that you understand what it says.

Only a few optical practitioners will state that their goal is to help children eventually get out of glasses. If you discover one of these gems, you are ahead in the game. Most practitioners will want to give the child a full 100 percent prescription that corrects his eyesight to 6/6 (20/20). If you are serious about doing my program, ask the receptionist on the phone if the doctor is willing to give the child an undercorrected pair of glasses. Patronization is a clear message to find a different practitioner.

If you discern that the first office is an ice cave, graciously bow out. Phone a different office and take yourself through the same process. If you feel comfortable with the service you are promised, go on to the next step.

When in the clinic be even more audacious. Ask the doctor to keep special records on your child. Is he willing to give you a discount price on regular three- or six-month visits so that an improvement in vision can be monitored and glasses reduced further? An optician in Singapore noticed that NVI students were rapidly dropping myopic correction. Delighted, he offered NVI students free eye exams as they improved their myopia. They paid only for their next pair of weaker lenses.

## Researching Surgery

Your child may be dealing with a turned eye—strabismus. Both behavioral optometrists and ophthalmologists love to treat strabismus, the first with glasses and visual training, the latter with surgery and possibly orthoptics. Studies have compared the success rate of these procedures. An article published by Nathan Flax and Robert Duckman, optometrists, shows vision training alone has a 76 percent cure rate.

When approaching an ophthalmic surgeon, use the preceding checklist, plus:

- What kind of anesthesia is used for the operation?
- What are the side effects of the anesthesia?
- What percentage of children have fusion after the operation?
- Would you kindly describe to me exactly what is done during the operation.
- Is there any follow-up check on the eyes and at what intervals?

- Do you recommend vision training instead of or after such an operation?

Some parents like to study textbooks. I was unable to obtain any information about strabismus operations from the ophthalmology department in Brisbane. It is not given out to people who are not enrolled as medical students.

If I could not get information for researching a book on the subject, what luck would an ordinary citizen have? I tried a different tactic. One of the NVI-trained optometrists in Sydney called the Department of Ophthalmology at Sydney University: She was told that information about textbooks would not be given to optometrists, only to medical doctors. She was able to order the desired book for me, in her name, from her own association.

The ophthalmology textbook eventually arrived. I suggest you order these books directly from the publishers, bypassing authoritarian roadblocks.

Educate yourself to make wise decisions about your child. Be a pest and ask annoying questions in the name of love. Your child's eyes are worth it!

# Obtaining and Using Transition Glasses

Members of the optical industry chant, "This child must wear his glasses or his eyes will get worse." This threat comes out of the minds of people who do not believe that vision can be improved through natural means. You will have to skirt this mind-set. Give a megaphone to the mousy voice that whispers, "But I wore glasses and my vision got worse."

If you choose to trust in the innate healing power of the mind and body, if you are willing to sacrifice the values of a society that schools its children into depression and burnout, then consider the following:

Prescription glasses lock eyes into the degree of correction. If a child relaxes for five minutes, his vision will be better. When he puts on full prescription glasses, his eyeballs must serve that prescription, just as ladies used to squeeze themselves into whalebone corsets. Signs that glasses are too strong are headaches and a feeling that your eyeballs are being pulled forward out of your face. Perhaps you've experienced this when picking up a new pair of prescription spectacles, and you've been told upon questioning, "Wear them, you will get used to it."

Your visual system will do its best to see clearly through glass that has too high a curve in it—the curve that was determined when you were seeing at your worst under test conditions.

Eyes need room to play, to change, especially when glasses are used. NVI

Myopic blur circle

Hyperopic blur circle

No blur circle

Using pinholes to increase saccadic motion and relax eyes

students often progress backward through several pairs of Transition Glasses until they no longer need any correction.

The guidelines for Transition Glasses have been determined by driving requirements. This level of vision is also adequate for seeing the board at school and for reading. These "T-Glasses" allow the eyes and visual system room for improvement.

Since most children are not driving a car, an important alternative for T-Glasses is to use child-sized pin-hole spectacles. Pin-holes consist of opaque plastic blanks with rows of punched holes. They are not legal for driving if there is a restriction on your driver's license. There is no prescription involved with pin-holes, and the optical industry is bypassed. Its members have used their political clout in the United States and Australia to try to keep pin-holes off the market.

The pin-holes have some advantages over prescription glasses They are inexpensive compared with the gorgeous frames sold by opticians and optometrists. They require no visits to the clinic. Vision can improve using the pin-holes until they are no longer needed.

Other pluses with the pin-holes include the fact that it is difficult to stare through them. The fly-eye effect, of looking through many holes, requires that the child keep his head moving slightly, thus releasing the back of his neck and inducing scanning rather than staring. Edging with the Magic Nose Pencil (page 75) through the pin-holes produces brilliant clarity. The marketing of pin-holes as a device that will improve eyesight by itself is misleading. Changing visual habits is what results in naturally clear vision, but the pin-holes can be a useful tool in the meantime.

However, you may not be able to find pin-holes, or for some other reason, your child may need to wear prescription T-Glasses. In this case take the following guidelines to your optometrist or opthalmologist.

## Prescription Guidelines

Transition Glasses should correct the child's vision to a "blurry" 6/12 (20/40), both eyes together for distance and close. The amount of correction in the glasses will vary with each child.

Kindly remove if possible all correction for astigmatism. If it cannot be removed completely, reduce it as much as possible. Please do not leave in the glasses correction for astigmatism less than one-half diopter. Astigmatism is one of the easiest refractive errors to erase (see chapter 15).

No tint, antiglare coating, or UV block in the glasses please (the discussion about UV light and sunglasses for children is in chapter 9).

Don't use prisms to force turning eyes to straighten. Games will be done to foster the alignment and eventual fusing of the two eyes (see chapter 16 on strabismus and chapter 17 on fusion).

Buy plastic rather than metal frames. A metal strip running horizontally across the bridge of the nose short-circuits the governing meridian, affecting posture and brain function. As soon as your child is seeing better than 6/12 (20/40) through the Transition Glasses, it is time to weaken them again. This time span can vary from two weeks to six months.

The governing meridian. The arrows show direction of life-energy flow.

# 4

# Parent Power and Home Science

## Two Views of Parents

### How Doctors See Parents: Parents Are Dumb

Parents do not know and do not want to know anything about science. Therefore parents should be discouraged from thinking for themselves. If they do ask questions about vision, they should be given answers that will fit their level of ignorance and disinterest. Parents must be trained in school and through the media to obey the suggestions of authority figures. Parents must be discouraged from attempting to influence their child's poor vision in any way by telling them that such efforts would be useless or harmful. Parents should be constantly advised to make their children wear glasses and sunglasses all the time by whatever means possible.

Parents must not be asked for their opinion about the child's condition, as they are not trained to detect or recognize problems. Involving the parent in the child's diagnosis could lead to wasting time and delaying necessary medical intervention.

Parents must be told that their child will fall behind in school and be miserable in the classroom if steps are not taken for early detection and treatment with surgery or glasses. Everyone rightfully regrets it if a child falls behind her peers in academic achievement.

Parents will only act to the benefit of their child through fear.

## My View: Parents Are Wise

Given the right tools and knowledge, parents are capable of helping their children to better vision within the home and family setting.

Parents are both rational and intuitive. Their love for their children when supported by appropriate ideas leads them to intelligent and effective action.

Parents are creative thinkers whose main goal for their children is health and happiness. Parents are brave beings whose hearts and minds are open to alternative and fresh avenues to healing. Parents are capable of overcoming their own fears and doubts in the face of discouragement and criticism.

Parents should be encouraged to ask questions. This helps the doctors, teachers, friends, and family arrive at the most effective approach to healing the child's vision problem.

Parents who have not yet realized all this about themselves will do so readily when given the opportunity.

# Healing the Parent

When you, as a parent, play vision games with your child, you will be healing both the child within yourself and your own vision. You will experience the absolute joy of discovering yourself, instead of falling into the discouragement and depression that most adults experience. The bespectacled mother who brings her child to NVI and says, "Just fix my kid. It's too late for me" is expressing self-contempt.

Lynn Bernard, a certified NVI teacher, contributed her experience:

> Meredith means "Gift from the sea/see." To truly appreciate the effectiveness of using Natural Vision Improvement techniques during pregnancy and labor, one must know about the birth of Meredith's older sister. I birthed her with the very stressful mind-set of "This is a hard, scary thing to do." At every decision point I took the "safe conventional route." As a result her birth was an agonizing twenty-nine hours; every intervention made to protect the baby actually endangered her, causing further complications, the ramifications of which are still unraveling today.
>
> With Meredith I had been freed of the demon of trying to please everyone else at my own expense. Because I was no longer in abject emotional pain I was able to feel with my heart what was right and see through the chicaneries of convention. I had always felt that home birth would be best for me. The

Black Earth Mother that I dreamed in a Palming session during the NVI instructor training reappeared during Meredith's birth as my black midwife. I studied with Jeannie Parvati-Baker to train my mind to believe birth is ecstasy.

During the pregnancy I played NVI "Painting Pictures" many times. The night before the birth I painted a virgin forest in Virginia. The emerald green fern forest glimmered in my imagination. When the midwife arrived the next cloudy morning I was very dilated. During one contraction I was running through that virgin forest, feeling the bracken under my feet, smelling the pine, hearing the birds, and finally transforming myself into a white moth. I flew into a sunbeam. From that moment on every contraction was cruising. I went into the tub. There was a cassette on called *Sojourn*. Later, as I examined the cassette I realized my thought patterns had followed the title of each song. I was very much in tune with my surroundings. I cried and asked my husband's forgiveness for rejecting his love so often. I was at ten centimeters in twenty minutes. This was seven hours of ecstasy. Every instant was gratifying, until I had to push. Then I clutched and had to be alone in a dark space. I remembered down to body level how wrong everything had gone at Frances's birth.

[Several hours of labor later.] When Meredith was born the sun broke through the clouds, the sky cleared, and the earth warmed. We sunned ourselves outside that afternoon.

Even with such a tremendously beautiful birth there were complications. First Meredith refused to breathe. Then she refused to nurse. Almost immediately we found her eye was turned. We gave her a homeopathic remedy and did lots of Bird Swings together. Her eye righted itself within two weeks. Thank God Frances had no such problem. I would have totally rejected her, such had been my close-mindedness.

I love both my daughters. It's so hard to explain this experience simply. I would love for all women to have their minds so freed that they could enjoy birth as I did or more. Some people think they can just hear or read someone saying, "Oh, my birth was ecstatic!" and assume theirs will be too. Well, it took a lot of practice to get to that point. The victims who came to me with recriminations, "Let me tell you it was no fun for me"—they didn't even try to have fun. They didn't ask about spirituality, mind-set, breathing, or nutrition. I offer this story not as a boast but so that your minds may be opened and so that you may see.

# Home Science As the New Authority

The vast majority of people, including the optical industrialists, accept the mechanical response to vision because this is what they learned first. What you learned as a child and young adult in school is your truth—unless disease, disaster, or sudden insight forces you to abandon the old pattern. Ordinary life does not usually pack the wallop needed to crack the initial mold; in fact, it is constantly being reinforced by our social mirrors.

The mechanical response is easiest, for it uses only 5 percent of our life energy and thumps any challengers with an iron fist. Yet life energy never dies; when thwarted it makes trouble in the eyes. Regard your child's vision development as an opportunity to directly experience life energy with its inherent up and downs. Make your own experience the highest science and top-dog authority.

To gain "proof" that your loving actions and application of natural healing do have an effect, you have to be the scientist. Science is not meant to be a cage in which ideas grow stale. True scientists observe without prejudice. They experiment with both tried and untried methods. They also document their findings and share them with others.

Your direct experience is added to the growing pool of wisdom that emphasizes what I call "personal science"—an internal knowing that goes beyond anger or rebellion. In the past thirty years gentle birthing methods, breast-feeding, and alternative health care have been growing in this way in spite of the opposition from doctors and governments. Make *your* personal-science contribution. Give yourself the opportunity and the praise. Respect your own experience. Think for yourself. It's not a case of either NVI or the doctors. You can choose any combination you like, utilizing the services of orthodox medical care and the actions described in this book. Bridge the gap in your own mind and come out of the illusion of isolation that parents experience when faced with an abnormal diagnosis of their child's vision.

Use the following guidelines to channel your observations, intuition, questions, and answers into written form. This data will be of joy to you and your children when they later ask about their formative years. Twenty-year-old eyes light up when age-two stories and photos come out. You will be able to stand solid in your sharing when you look back and assess the effectiveness of your loving and healing actions, whether anyone else validated them or not!

# Keeping a Vision Journal

I know even keeping a shopping list is difficult enough. Many of us are wounded writers after being graded in school on our fledgling compositions. How do we get ourselves to write down the precious moments of insight and small landmarks? Keep your Vision Journal simple and easily accessible. Here are a few tips:

> Buy a clipboard. Hang it on a nail in the kitchen with a pen attached, or place it near the dining table where you can sit down and write.
> Buy a colorful binder and a hole puncher.
> Keep lots of plain paper in a drawer to put on your clipboard.
> Keep some crayons handy for the time when the child wants to sit on your lap and draw pictures as her contribution to the journal.

# Your Own History

### Write Your History, As a Mother or Father

Close your eyes and take three deep breaths.

Pretend you are talking to me or your best friend. This writing is free-form. All your critics are vacationing on an island in the South Pacific. Write the following history and place it in your notebook:

- My attitude toward life and my lifestyle before this child was born was . . .
- My feeling toward children was . . .
- The conception of this child was . . .

Describe the nature of the pregnancy:

- The physical circumstances, in my body and in the environment, were . . .
- I was eating . . .
- My emotional state was . . .

Write about the nature of this child's birth:

- The place.
- The people.
- The mother's experience.

- The infant's state.
- Do you see any possibility of congenital eye problems relating to the birthing style?
- Were there mechanical stresses, for example, prolonged labor, forceps delivery?
- Were there chemical stresses, for example, anesthesia, smoking, toxemia? Were silver nitrate drops used? Were there toxic substances in or around the home such as mothballs or pesticides?
- What time of day was this child born?
- What were the lighting conditions at this child's birth?
- Has one or have both of the parents used any medical drugs such as cortisone or antidepressants, or any recreational drugs?
- What was the medical history of the parents and grandparents?

# This Wonderful Child

Describe your current living conditions:

- The place, the people.
- The child's responses.
- Your diet; the child's diet.
- Sleeping arrangements.
- What's happening with eyes and vision?
- What did you do in response to these circumstances?
- Have you used any suggested NVI activities? If so, which ones were you able to use? How often, approximately?
- What changes have you noticed as a result of your own actions to support and remedy this wonderful child's general and visual situation? List changes in yourself, changes in your child.

If your child is already older and a lot of history has flowed under the bridge, may I suggest you use a timeline as shown below. Put the key events regarding the child to the left of the line. Put your subjective feelings and thoughts to the right of the line. For example:

| Event and age | My thoughts and feelings |
|---|---|
| Bettina is born. | My cup floweth over. |
| At six months I notice her right eye is turning in. | I'm worried. Everyone says, "Take her to the eye specialist," who says, "Come back in six months. There's nothing you can do in the meantime. She may grow out of it." |
| At eighteen months we go to Baby Play Group together one morning a week. | I'm nervous about what the other parents think of me. |
| | I love being able to talk with the other mothers about the children. |

# Doctors' Reports and Prescriptions

Attach an envelope to your journal and place all doctors' reports in the envelope. Write down your response and describe your child's reaction to the visits to the clinic.

Add the doctors' medical treatments and recommendations, a vaccination history, and accounts of healing crises (illness). If you are not able to understand the doctor or optometrist's report, ask her to put it in plain English, as if you need it for a trip overseas. Make sure you understand the report enough to explain your child's condition to someone else.

The following example shows you how to read a prescription.

The number in the "sphere" box designates the strength of the lenses for either hyperopia or myopia. A minus (-) before the number will be for myopia; a plus (+) before the number signifies a hyperopic correction. A plus lens magnifies everything you see through it; a minus lens reduces images. The cylinder and axis refer to an astigmatism correction.

The numeral -2.5 in the right eye "sphere" box means the child is myopic in that eye. She needs a lens with a focusing strength of two and one-half diopters. Window glass has no diopters. One diopter is the amount of curve in a lens that will focus light to a point one meter (about one yard) away. The boxes for cylinder and axis are used only if there is astigmatism correction. This child has been given one diopter of astigmatism correction at an angle (axis) of 15 degrees. The axis is the angle of astigmatism. (Turn to chapter 15 to understand and resolve astigmatism.) If the sphere numeral were +2.5, this child would be hyperopic.

| | SPH (sphere) | CYL (cylinder) | AXIS |
|---|---|---|---|
| Right Eye | -2.5 | -1 | x15 |
| Left Eye | | | |

The following pages can be photocopied. Use them to organize your Natural Vision Improvement games.

## Planning Your Vision Games

Today's date_____Child's name_____is now age_____

The doctor says_____vision problem is:

_____

_____

_____

_____

From chapter(s)_____I find that we could be doing the following activities:

_____

_____

_____

_____

For the last_____month(s) we have actually been doing the following vision games:

_____

_____

_____

_____

This is what I think and how I feel about the whole situation:

_____

_____

_____

_____

What do we want to accomplish over the next three months?

_____

_____

_____

_____

_____

These are the ways I want to go about it:

_____

_____

_____

_____

_____

Send your story to:

> Natural Vision Improvement Center Pty. Ltd.
> 12 Crystal Waters
> Maleny, Queensland, Australia 4552

Please send photocopies of your data pages.

Do add your feelings and thoughts. They will be read and appreciated.

Please mark the appropriate box:

☐ I wish this report to be kept confidential.

☐ Our story may be shared with others.

Signed_____Date_____

Address_____

_____

# 5

# A Child Grows Vision

## What Is a Child?

What is your definition of a child? Are children miniature adults waiting to get big enough to work in an office? Are they extensions of parental bloodlines and egos? Or are they incarnated droplets of spirit?

Is childhood special in itself, or is it just a hallway leading to the living room? Should we stand back in awe at the metamorphosis taking place or hurry things along?

If children are adults in embryo, then keep your sights on the future adult and his place in society. The school system prepares children for adulthood in a competitive society. Young Joe will one day be supporting a family; he needs a good job. Teach him how to use a computer early. Don't let him wander by the creek. In this camp a child's vision problem is regarded solely as a blockage to performance.

This attitude toward children and education is antiquated. Management philosopher Charles Handy, author of *The Age of Paradox*, predicts that in ten years people will be holding down that "good job" for twenty-five, not forty-five, years. He encourages workers to stop thinking exclusively about careers and to develop their lives like artists' portfolios. Everyone is advised to give equal value to wages, leisure time, community service, and personal development.

## Is Childhood Special?

Is childhood a magical time in itself? A few adults remember an ineffable glow from their childhood and the fullness of what they saw. These people look at a child and see a snowflake gleaming with uniqueness. They trust that the child contains everything he needs to grow, heal, and be self-sufficient, instead of worrying about how he will carve his path.

The desire to recapture, to study, and to acknowledge that there is something special about childhood must be honored before it is too late. Samuel Silverstein, a science teacher, writes:

> I believe that all children live in two worlds, both at the same time, interlocked with each other; the ordinary world that we all see as children move about in daily life, and a "hidden world" in which they are in contact with God's presence . . . "a hidden world," which is available to children all the time in early childhood, but after the age of eight or so starts disappearing. Eventually it becomes mostly a "lost world"—the lost world of childhood. As adults, unless we have the ability to recall those experiences of childhood, we will have at best only hazy memories of what once occurred.

## The Self-Regulated Child

Self-regulation allows the child himself to determine when he fits into adult schedules and demands. It also means allowing the child freedom of choice wherever possible, to change, learn, and grow in his own patterns. It is freedom but not license.

I was proud of the fact that my baby at eight weeks was sleeping through the night. I simply could not fathom why the young mother visiting my parents was waking her baby up at night to give him his four-hour bottle. That's one difference between the self-regulated and the other-regulated child.

There are also times when things look good to the parent but the child says no for her own reasons. When Carina was five I found a school for her that I loved. The teachers were alternative, the kids cute. There was a garden with large trees. Carina attended for two weeks. On the third Monday she refused to get off the couch and into the car. I phoned the teacher. "Carina is playing games with you," she said.

My respect for Carina's perception was intact. I couldn't see what was wrong with the place. She could not explain it to me. We went together to find a different school.

The child becomes the teacher in this arena. To experience the self-regulated child (I suspect one is already resident in your house), stop everything you are doing and thinking. Look at your child. Ask him what is happening, how he feels, and what he would like to do about his eyesight. The response could be verbal or silent. Present him with alternatives. His choice may not please you directly, but each new development of the child's abilities will show you exactly when and how to play a vision game. The following overview will alert your mind to those opportunities.

## Babies Are the Real Experts

The philosophy of treating, nurturing, and helping children has been a battlefield for centuries.

Only now are the experts becoming clever enough to ask the child. In the past the observations of the mothers were seldom given any credence. This lack of interaction with the concerned parties resulted in some barbaric and unfeeling methods of dealing with children and their problems.

"There's no use dangling rattles in front of the baby's eyes," a Melbourne ophthalmologist told a mother with a cross-eyed baby. "There's no perception there yet." This fellow was suffering from knowledge gap. Science has changed. By monitoring the infant's heart rate, galvanic skin response, head movements, eye movements, and eager sucking, psychologists discovered that babies are sensing more than they are telling. They discovered what mothers have suspected all along. Infants are born with intelligence and a whole lot of perception. Six-hour-old babies are already noting the changing expressions on mom's face and tracking triangles.

But please, parents, don't run out and buy a computer for your six-month-old child. Trust the pacing of the innate, the native intelligence. It comes with the package. Some of the babies being trained in the cradle to read are doing calculations in the sand at age three instead of playing with pail and shovel. It used to be that myopia began at age seven. Owing to early left-brain schooling, myopia is now appearing at age four. Presenting a task before the child's motor development and brain integration are ready to perform that task may be counterproductive.

## Stages of Growth

The following guide is given so that you may start vision games suitable to your child's level of development.

An important hint about static timetables: If your child lags several months behind a milestone, or you feel in your heart that he is exhibiting distress, then take him to a practitioner for examination and diagnosis. But don't worry unduly if your child is tardy. The phases of childhood depicted on the timelines that follow are averages. Many children walk at nine months. Bright-eyed, sturdy Aerro decided to walk at twenty months after becoming a virtuoso crawler. Most children are taught to read at ages six or seven. My son was more interested in swinging from the trees at that age. At ten he proclaimed he was ready to learn reading. We spent two weeks doing Cross-Crawl, turning his reading errors into hilarious playacting. He asked for special attention at school. Within two weeks he was reading fluently. The child who regulates his own learning becomes a master.

Notice how in normal development phases children enter chaos and reorganize in a six-month rhythm. Negative symptoms are natural during the fall-apart phase. It's meant to be a temporary crisis. Stopping in a phase leads to chronic problems; then children get stuck in visual blur or turned eyes. Using the activities in this book may help you sail through chaos and crises.

A certified Natural Vision Improvement instructor who works with children may reside near you. If not, you may wish to take the instructor training program yourself and/or attend one of the Parent and Child Playcamps.

Never force a child to do a game. Play the game with him. If he snubs you, play the game by yourself. He will be watching out of the corner of his eye.

## Infants Are Sensing: Birth to Four Months

The "competent infant" is a new catchword in psychology. The visual system develops rapidly. These infants are no longer empty boards to be written on, nor are they "bundles of reflexes." Newborns are astounding in their ability to perceive visually and to respond to stimulus. Social contact and visual stimulation are most important through:

Holding and rhythmic swinging
Creating an interesting visual environment (use chapter 8)
The rocking chair and the Bird Swing (page 80)
Making sounds together: humming, crooning, singing, babbling, and especially yawning
Introducing kicking and batting toys (page 73)

At birth the baby's peripheral sighting range is 30 degrees to the sides. At seven weeks he sees objects at 45 degrees. By five months babies can tell the difference between a cube and a wedge.

Distance and depth perception emerge between three and six months. As soon as an infant begins to blink or reach toward an approaching object you can introduce Near-Far Swings. This is useful for babies with turned eyes (refer to chapter 16). Do Near-Far movements with a colorful object held in your hand. Move the object in all directions.

It is normal for an infant to alternate looking with one eye, then the other. Using both eyes together takes a big jump between sixteen and twenty-one weeks. An infant born with a turning eye shows no acuity difference between his two eyes until he is twenty weeks old. If there is no stimulation to the brain receiving the message from the turning eye, acuity begins to drop. This fact causes some surgeons to insist that babies born with strabismus be operated on before the age of six months.

Other therapies can be used even at this early stage. Osteopathic and chiropractic consultation with a practitioner specializing in young children is available. Gentle manipulation of skull bones could repair any mechanical trauma from a difficult or forceps birth.

It is never too late to recover lost ground. Even if brain cell columns in the visual cortex have not developed properly, the body can still organize itself in a normal manner. Parents can help the rebalancing process further with regular exercises such as those found in this book or provided by an Educational Kinesiology practitioner or at a developmental play group such as Gymboree.

## Older Babies Explore: Eight to Twelve Months

Newly hatched humans are now moving from the wriggly fish stage to the independent quadruped stage. Personal status is growing. When crawling begins, a spirit of exploration appears that is insatiable. The index finger makes itself evident, pointing here and there. Touching what we see is a profound experience.

### Games to Play
### (favoring the phoria if need be; see chapter 16, on strabismus):
Peek-a-boo.
Practice walking (after he's stood by himself).
Point to the opposite foot with the opposite hand.
Finger plays and songs.
Ball games of all sorts.

Push a ball and crawl after it.
"Let's go find something."
Nesting boxes.
Continue Mirror Swings for turning eyes (page 179).
Bang and blink.
"Let's attach toys to strings and pull them to us."

## The Emergent Toddler Imitates

### Games to Play

"Get social with a group" ball games.
"Monkey see, monkey does, laugh your head off."
"See what's up high, see what's down there."
Buttons sewn on things, buckles, zippers.
Put large bright objects in a special vision box.
"Let's take the hat on and off."
Finger plays: for example, patty-cake.
"Now you run and hide and I will come after you."
Sit in a circle while baby walks from lap to lap, with a hug at each stop.

When walking begins, the conquering of space takes top priority. Toddlers are now interested in the fate of moving objects. The expansion of the mind is outward. Use a trip in the car or a walk, perhaps with an eye patch on, to explore textures and things that move with appropriate verbal signals. Use the words *look* and *see*.

## Advanced Toddlers Pretend

Toddlers are now learning voluntary control of muscles—potty training, for example. Babbling turns into recognizable words. Manners, morals, and emotions are discussed and enforced. Boundaries are established. Self-regulation does not mean abuse.

The toddler's two-sided capacities grow. Some scientists say that between the ages of three and five years the dominant side of hand, foot, eye, and ear will be established. Dr. Arnold Gesell says this takes place between ages five and eight.

### Games to Play

Build towers and make them crash.
Wrap things up in paper.

Water play.
Mimic sounds, gestures, faces.
Play with wheels and whirlies.
Put small objects rather than big ones in the vision box.
Hide-and-find games.
Cross-Crawl dancing followed by other two-person sports.

At age *two and one-half* the child is into extremes and dualism: on and off, here and there, you and I, front and back, yes and no, asleep and awake. Intense contact with people and objects is necessary for the drive to a higher level of development. He needs "hands-on" contact with all things and people, rather than sitting alone in front of a TV set.

The physicality of this age group means that every adult and caregiver has to get off his or her bottom and move. No use yelling from a distance; the exercise will do you good. Interacting in a friendly physical fashion will relax your muscles and delight the child. Tickle and massage him instead of swatting him.

The "tiny tyrant" may appear. This is his left-brain practice at being sure and right about his possessions and his territory. This behavior is a protection and may become ritualized so that things are "right there." Crossed eyes can appear where they weren't before. This is a perfect time to bring in directional vision games.

## Three- and Four-Year-Olds Organize

### Games to Play

Matching and lotto games.
Name landmarks when walking.
"Let's pretend" while palming.
Make things out of clay and name them.

At *three and a half*, new pressures arise. Children will say, "Don't look at me." Earlier brain integration falls apart once more for the purpose of reorganizing on a higher level. It's necessary. Have you not noticed this in your own adult life? Grown-ups hate to fall apart. Children do not judge disintegration. They allow the intelligence of their life energy to put their body and mind back together.

While in disintegration, this child will see only one side of the story. His timing is faulty. He will drop a glass of water. Divergence may appear in the eyes, and he may use the words, "I can't see."

### Actions to Take

Read a book and play Nuclear Vision games with the pictures.

Palm and pretend how you want things to be.

Act out what you imagine together. Become the lion and roar.

Make up funny names for things and people.

Use imaginary companions to sort out negative and positive emotions, then bring them together with Melting Beach Balls (page 119).

At *age four*, both sides of the brain are talking to each other again. Self-confidence, expansiveness, and fluidity reappear as these right-brain abilities kick in.

### Games to Play

Play vision games with large objects such as a yardstick or meter stick.

Engage in space and muscles action: skipping, climbing under chairs and tables, making a playhouse out of a table with a cloth over it.

Put on improvised dramas with animal characters.

Explore the sky, the ocean, the world, while Palming.

Use round letters with Painting White on homemade eye charts from chapter 12.

Make large drawings with big crayons and paint.

Spend lots of time outdoors with your vision games.

## Five-Year-Olds Create

This cool person is interested in fact and reality. He has things well in hand. The left-brain theme of this period makes ending things easier than starting things.

### Games to play

Draw and trace with the Magic Nose Pencil (page 79).

Copy and color (houses and homes are themes).

Start Painting White around letters, numbers, and animal shapes while jumping on the trampoline (page 135).

Do Bird Swings and Nuclear Vision games: in books, in the kitchen, outdoors (pages 80 and 88–93).

Put letters with vertical lines on the child's eye chart.

Set up a walking board (pages 219).

## Six-Year-Olds Question

Right-brain shifts of mood and lack of follow-through reappear. The child's eyes may not want to work together. He may become ill and fatigued. Pressure about having to attend school and adhere to strict rules at the table should be eased. He may dawdle, refuse, rebel, vacillate. He may lose his place when reading. Standing up in front of the class to read aloud could become a lifetime trauma. All this is normal to the growth process. So far, the pendulum has been swinging in approximately six-month intervals through right- and left-brain qualities. The intervals may become longer as the child moves into the primary school.

### Games to Play

Lots of Cross-Crawl dancing, yoga, stretching, and body images.

Space questions: how big? how long? how far?

Oblique lines, for example, the letter *K* (letters with slanted lines can be drawn and used on the eye chart).

Share beautiful things: sunsets, rainbows, clouds.

Vision games of pursuit-and-follow, for example, Near-Far Swings.

Elves, fairies, and dinosaurs may appear while Palming.

## Seven-Year-Olds Build

The thinker appears. He often talks to himself. He may withdraw and need a special cubby house or a nest in the garden in a pile of mown grass. Feelings are being examined. Don't be late, and don't fail. Fantasies of packing a suitcase and leaving home arise; a map may be requested. Repetition is satisfying.

### Games to Play

Play ball games again. Buy a bat and a softball.

Do Nuclear Vision games to find the center of his mind and visual field (pages 88–93).

Listening is now important, so Palm with music, picking out the different instruments.

Listen to stories.

Draw and erase, then repeat the process.

## Eight- to Ten-Year-Olds Intellectualize

These children are competent and their brains integrated except when emotional, chemical or body stresses arise. Clubs and groups are organized. They love to put on plays and shows, assemble toys and models. Collections of stamps and coins or stuffed animals fill shelves and drawers. Guessing what is happening from sight and hearing is enjoyed.

### Games to play

"I spy" vision games, card games with eye patches.

Make vision tests and visits to the doctor into scripts for plays.

Do lots of Painting White on self-made eye charts (pages 129 and 135).

Play games with trails, tunnels, and treasure maps.

Explore the seven emotions with dramatic stories (page 118).

Use comics and graphic novels for tracing with the Magic Nose Pencil.

Discuss motion pictures and TV programs while Palming.

Make eye charts with roads and pathways leading to letters and numerals (page 129).

Part 2

# Keen Eyesight for Every Child

# 6

# Your Child's Electric Body

## Use Reflex Points to Help Vision

Mechanically, a reflex is an immediate involuntary response called forth by stimulating a particular area of the body. If an ant bites your toe, your eyes will immediately search for the source of the pain. Your foot will lift up by itself. This is an example of nerve reflex action. There are several kinds of reflex pathways in the human body.

The stomach meridian runs from the foot to the eye and ear on both sides of the body.

In Chinese medicine, acupuncture needles are placed along meridian flow lines to ensure that chi (life energy) is flowing in a balanced way through the whole body. Meridians can also be stimulated by acupressure massage or by simply holding a reflex point. Meridians reflex directly to organs and glands.

If you've ever gulped down freezing-cold ice cream and felt a pain at your forehead, you were overstimulating the stomach meridian. The pain was trying to tell you something about eating ice-cold food: it damages the stomach lining.

Meridians and reflex points are part of the body's electrical system. Imagine the human body as a Christmas tree draped with chains of colored lightbulbs. The display is invisible, but it is still there. Physical malfunction or emotional distress is a signal that the lighting system needs attention.

Holding reflex points puts the plug into the electrical socket. Electrons stream through the wires, up and down. Around the tree red, green, and gold areas of light radiate. *Ohhh*, everyone sighs, and feels different. Your fingers and hands are the electrical sockets full of electromagnetic energy. Contacting specific points on your child's body reestablishes and increases the flow of primal life energy.

You can use the reflex response to balance and restore life energy flow to the eyes themselves and to the visual brain, where 80 percent of vision takes place.

The effect of holding a point is immediate. I have chosen points that will be easy for you to use daily while interacting with your child. Hugging, holding, cuddling, stroking, tickling, and rocking are instinctive acts. Learning the following points will give your natural caresses a healing tone.

In the 1930s, Frank Chapman, an American osteopath, discovered subtle pulses on the head that he named *neurovascular reflexes*. The rhythm of these points is unrelated to heartbeat. It may be a primitive pulsation of capillaries in the skin. Hold these points lightly; the effect is improved blood circulation to related muscles and organs. I have chosen three neurovascular points on the skull that connect directly to eyesight.

The areas to stimulate on the back are called *neurolymphatic reflexes*. These two shoulder points foster lymph flow to the eyes and related muscles. The third, lower-back, point is used if your child has a turning eye. Nerve reflexes for the eyes are also found on the fingers and toes. This lore came from ancient India.

# Preverbal Language

Emotional as well as physical messages are transmitted through the reflex points. Holding the points is like turning on a radio broadcast along with the Christmas tree lights. This broadcast is not coming through in any spoken language. It is a language that hides nothing and cannot lie.

Most adults have forgotten the unspoken language. Parents desperately ask their screaming baby, "What's wrong with you? Do you just want attention?" By going quiet within and assuming your hunches are correct, your ability to decipher this language will sharpen.

I have named the reflex areas according to broadcasts heard while working with NVI students. If you are holding points and massaging older children, the suppressed feeling that blocked a channel may show itself. Referring to chapter 11 will give you more ideas for unblocking rivers of sadness and volcanoes of anger.

We do not wish to deny "negative" expressions but to have compassion for the difficulty of experiencing them. For example, when holding the "Peace Point" you could say out loud, "I know you are feeling overwhelmed by life." Once the negative is fully acknowledged and experienced, the intelligence that governs our healing process will assert itself. The "positive" expressions come in their turn: "I know you are capable."

Reflex points
for vision

# What about "Born with It"?

Babies and children are marvelously open, both physically and emotionally. You can start relating to these points from the first few days out of the womb. The less time the blockage has to establish itself, the less time it takes to reactivate the flow of energy through a reflex point. But start any time. You may simply have more logs to remove from the creek if the child is already seventy. Even then it is the person's willingness to change that counts, not how high the logjam is.

Even though life energy may be blocked, it is never destroyed. When it is blocked in one area, it takes itself to some other part of the body and annoys us with an ache or a twitch, and eventually with an abnormality or disease.

Life energy flows through genetic bloodlines. You inherit a landscape. Think about the flowing creek, whose source is a bottomless spring. If you dam the creek, the water will still flow even though it's not moving according to the ideal plan. It may form numerous small rivulets. It could turn your garden into a marsh. Erosion could start on the hillside. Perhaps your ancestors cut down all the trees to build houses and cooking fires. The result of that action can be inherited, not necessarily in a mathematically genetic way like hemophilia, but as a tendency or latent weakness. This helps us understand how babies can exhibit crossed eyes or come out of the womb heading in a particular direction. Head them off at the pass and reassert the proper landscape, the proper setting for maximum recovery.

All energy blockages are attached to an experience of some kind, to a memory that may be stored unconsciously deep in the brain or in DNA. With someone who is forty years old we might have to hold the eye points for one and a half hours before the hidden memory of almost drowning on the beach becomes conscious. On a baby of three months, holding your fingertips gently on the point for one minute at a time will reestablish the proper flow of the creek. We may wonder if the child also goes to the movies while we hold her reflex points. If she is asleep and we notice the REMs under her eyelids, we know she is dreaming. May these dreams cleanse and release family patterns, no matter how they were created or manifested.

# Point Holding

The method: place your fingertips on the points shown with a feather touch, holding them for at least as long as it takes you to hum a favorite tune or sing one of the lullabies in this chapter. These songs have been especially composed for this purpose.

Hold each point or pair of points in the *order shown*.

How often? If your baby's eyes and vision are *normal*, you can use these points occasionally. If your baby's eyes are *crossed*, or there is an indication of *abnormal vision*, hold these points every day while you are feeding or cuddling, or while the child is asleep. With older children have a "Hold a Point Party" where you come together for a few minutes of relaxation. Older children can hold these points on themselves and on each other.

What to feel for: After you become relaxed with the idea of using your own hands for healing and after finding comfortable body positions for holding the points, you may detect a tiny pulsation through your fingers. One mother described the sensation as a "tingling warmth" and a "tiny burst of energy." If you don't perceive this pulse, hold the points anyway and be open to noticing it in the future.

## The Peace Point

**Emotion/thought:**

| Negative | Positive |
|---|---|
| I'm overwhelmed. | I am at peace. |

The Peace Point is at the crown of the head. This area is called the *anterior fontanel* on a newborn. The skull bones will not have grown together completely and you can easily feel the infant's heartbeat at this point. Move your finger to the very top of this area; your finger is a feather. Imagine the life energy rising out of this point like a fountain. The word *fontanel* comes from old French, meaning "a little fountain." We want a little fountain of energy to spring up continually from the top of the child's head.

The emotional significance of this point is peacefulness versus feeling overwhelmed. As you hold the point, observe your own thoughts and body sensations. Write down your observations about feeling overwhelmed by life and its demands. See if you and the child come out of this gentle experience with a greater sense of calmness.

The Peace Point

## Loving Support Points

**Emotion/thought:**

| Negative | Positive |
|---|---|
| Nobody wants/loves me. | Everything and everyone loves me. |

At the base of the skull there are two indentations where the neck muscles attach to the skull. These are the muscles with which we nod "yes" to life. They are powerful points for communicating love into the body. Locate these two points on yourself first. See if they are tender. Find them on your child and hold them while you both relax. You could cradle her head while she is sleeping, contacting these two points with your thumb and middle finger. If she is older and will lie down for a while, sit at her head and hold these two points with the middle fingers of both hands.

Loving Support Points

Loving Support Points

The emotional theme at these points is the question of love and being wanted. As you contact this part of the head, observe the "theme park" of your thoughts. If this child for any reason of its own (or because it may have been picking up on your issues) is dealing with feeling unloved or unwanted, send in very clear messages aloud, in song, or in thought. Even crooning "You are loved, you are loved" in a singsong is releasing stress. "The trees love you. Your papa (mama) loves you." (Even if she's gone missing.) "The birdies love you. The sky loves you." You may end up with some hot tears in your own eyes.

## Angel Wing Points

### Emotion/thought

| Negative | Positive |
|----------|----------|
| I'm too weak. | I can do anything. |

These two points at the corners of the shoulder blades are sore on anyone with vision problems. The divine push, the joy of creating new things, turns into burdens as we grow older. The initial joy of going to school and learning turns into test stress and biting nails. This is the place from which our wings would sprout if we took ourselves lightly. Contact these points on the child by putting your two hands under the child's back from the top. Or alternately hold the points with the child on his tummy.

Angel Wing Points

Angel Wing Points

## Ouch Points

### Emotion/thought

| Negative | Positive |
|----------|----------|
| I'm hurting. | I'm taken care of. |

Massage and hold the Ouch Points on the fingers. When your child is older she can hold them on herself and sing the song on page 53 changing the "you are" to "I am."

Eyes

Eye reflexes on fingers

## Blindness Points

### Emotion/thought

| **Negative** | **Positive** |
|---|---|
| I don't want to see. | Seeing is loving. |
| I don't want to be seen. | |

Massage and hold these areas. If children sit cross-legged, they can hold these points themselves and sing.

1 **Inner eye**

2 **Eye muscles**

Eye reflexes on toes

## The Ugly Duckling Point

For turning eyes, do all the points given above, plus the Ugly Duckling Point.

### Emotion/thought

| **Negative** | **Positive** |
|---|---|
| I am ugly. | I am beautiful. |

Hold the point indicated for as long as you like. Let your thoughts and feelings drift through you. Simply observe them. Croon a little tune or chant, "I love you when you're an ugly duckling. I love you when you are a swan." When the child is old enough for Palming, tell the Ugly Duckling story (page 108).

Ugly Duckling Point

**YOU ARE LOVED**

*Words and Music by Elizabeth Ledger, Adapted by Donald Woodward*

*Gently*

You are  loved.. You are  loved   by the  flow-ers and the trees.

By the  birds  in the sky,_____ the   wind___ and the

sun._____ Mm-mm-mm-mm-mm._____ You are  loved.__ You are

loved.__ Your  moth-er loves  you._____ Mm-mm - mm-mm-mm-mm-mm.__

You   are   here   to  be  loved._____

## Tickle Zones

When the child is older and you are tumbling on the floor or bed together, the preceding points can turn into tickle spots. "Get you right in there!" The song "Eentsy Weentsy Spider" is appropriate here (see page 55). The spider lands on the place where stress is held and wriggles about, his agile feet releasing the giggles and the tightness.

Ugly Duckling reflex area on adult spine— fifth lumbar vertebra

## Massage Muscles Related to Eyesight

Massage has many benefits. It can erase traumas and help people through crises. Stress hormones picked up in the womb are deactivated by stroking a newborn's skin. This contact bonds offspring and parents. In the words of Frederick Leboyer, M.D., children are reassured that the world outside the womb is also "alive and warm, beating and friendly." Repeatedly experiencing that closeness is a pleasure that can transmute difficult births or illnesses. Otherwise some of us continue to battle with life.

Make massage a family habit. After coping with fears and tears, adults also need steely shoulder muscles released. Helping others with massage and massaging oneself become as natural as yawning and breathing. Loosening neck and shoulders is helpful before writing a paper or after a fatiguing performance. Through the handy aid of massage, children learn that relaxation is possible under all circumstances.

Muscles are tied into the eyes through the "Christmas tree reflex network." Two pairs of muscles that tie directly into the visual system are the *trapezius* and the *back neck flexors*. The feet and hands may also be massaged, giving special attention to the eye points on the fingers and toes.

Everybody gets a trapezius massage.

## A Whole Baby/Child Massage

Put some old towels on the dining table or a mat on the floor. (Beds are usually too low and too soft for massage.) With a bowl of fresh olive or vegetable oil nearby, lay the baby or child down on her tummy to massage her feet for two or three minutes, then proceed with the whole foot and leg. Make sure you maintain a posture that's easy on your back.

Massage options:

- through clothing or undressed
- with oil from the kitchen, scented or not
- using aromatherapy (suggested fragrance: orange)
- with music or without music

Massage your child at least once a week, more often if possible. Newborn and infant massage is recommended every day. Take every unplanned opportunity to release your child's muscles. It will tranquilize you as well.

## Massage for the Trapezius

Trapezius muscle

Since the trapezius muscles are on the back, you can lay your child either on your lap or on the table on her tummy. Stroke with the flat of your hands up and down the whole back, sweeping in opposite directions with each hand. With the tips of your fingers make tiny circles up and down the spine just to the sides of the spinal processes (the little knobs where the spinal vertebrae stick out). Make a circle, lift your fingers, move to the adjacent area, make another circle. Continue in this fashion down to the tailbone and up to the base of the skull. Make these small circles all along the edge of the shoulder blade. This stimulates and relaxes the areas where the trapezius and neck flexors attach to the bones. Gently knead the top of the shoulders.

## Massage for Neck Flexors

Back neck flexors

With baby on her back, sit with her head between your legs. Reach under her neck and feel the neck muscles that run from the base of the skull down into the upper back. Using both hands together, pull up and toward you a few times. Start at the middle back and slowly proceed upward toward the head.

## Timetable for Massage and Point Holding

For any age you could do special-occasion full massages and include the eye points. Otherwise catch your child when you can, after learning the location of reflex points and muscles.

### Birth to One Year

Become accustomed to contacting the infant's head and body with your hands. Holding the baby in this gentle way will ease your fear about handling this tiny, delicate creature, and baby will receive the language of touch that tells her she is welcome and loved within the human family. Consult massage books and have a family massage day.

### Two to Five Years

You could hold eye reflex points at bedtime while listening to the adventures of the day or playing a story on cassette. Music would be good, or spontaneous storytelling. Children love to become little masseuses, trading massages with you.

### Five to Twelve Years

This age group likes to learn anatomy. Painting the muscles on each other with nontoxic paint or pens will lay out the ground. Consider short massages while sitting next to each other on the couch while watching TV with Transition Glasses and Magic Nose Pencils.

## No Right or Wrong

Are you anxious about whether you're doing things right or wrong? What's important is whether the energy is flowing. A person could do this whole method wrongly and still have successful changes take place because he or she did it with joy and unconditional love.

# 7

# Vision Is Alive and Well in the Brain

## Eyes Are Ruled by the Brain

Seeing takes place in the child's brain, not in his eyes. Any change in eyesight reflects something happening in the brain, either a shutdown or a turn-on.

Light beams come in the front of the eye and tickle the nerve cells of the retina. The nerve cells convert light into electricity and whiz the electrical messages deep into the brain via optic nerve cables. Along the way memos are sent to other parts of the body. Ears, hands, feet, saliva glands (if a tasty meal is beaming at you) are waiting for a buzz from the head office. Sometimes the memos don't arrive or they come in late. This results in confusion, visual blur, dyslexia.

Seeing takes place in the brain.

1  **Optic nerve cables**
2  **Front of eye**
3  **Retina**
4  **Switching stations send messages to the rest of the body**
5  **Visual brain at back of head processes signals from the eyes**

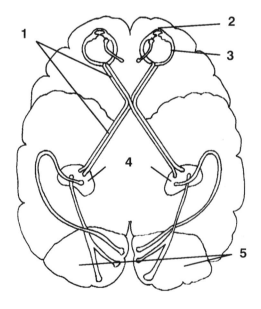

# Dueling Hemispheres

There are two major sides in the brain, two hemispheres. They are joined together by a communication bridge called the corpus callosum.

The behavior of people whose corpus callosum had been surgically severed has revealed that each hemisphere of the brain is responsible for certain human behaviors.

## The left hemisphere

- moving the right side of the body
- short-term memory, e.g., remembering a telephone number for ten seconds
- talking, thinking inside the head
- getting all the small close-up details
- trying and straining to move and to see
- learning new skills
- counting, calculating, worrying about being right or wrong

## The right hemisphere

- moving the left side of the body
- remembering things for a long time
- imagining, visualizing, making pictures in the mind
- moving and grooving through space
- grasping the situation as a whole
- automatic habits, e.g., riding a bike
- making music and keeping rhythm

This division of abilities in the brain is not cast in concrete. Both hemispheres are capable of playing any role. But it must be decided who will get the bright ideas and who will talk about them. If both sides of the brain try to speak at once, stuttering results. When six-year-old Wolfgang did not rattle off his times table fast enough, his father hit him. In order to escape this agony, Wolfgang forced his right hemisphere to make a place for seven times nine. If one hemisphere is injured, the other side may be called up for duty. There are even cases where people were born with only one hemisphere and still lived normally.

When we put ourselves under prolonged physical, mental, and/or emotional stress, our hemispheres stop talking to each other. We become of two minds, like a couple filing for divorce. One side says "Stay," the other side says "Go." One screams,

"You are not listening to me"; the other scornfully replies, "You're acting like a child." There may be clumsy or clever repartee but no reconciliation.

Brain battles relate directly to vision problems. The following chart shows the attributes related to vision and which side of the brain is in action.

| Left brain, "motor mind" | Right brain, "dream boat" |
| --- | --- |
| • muscles shorten, tighten | • muscles lengthen, relax |
| • seeing up close | • seeing in the distance |
| • watching the clock | • getting into it |
| • thinking and talking | • imagining and drawing |
| • staying alert | • calmness of mind |
| • trying, straining to see | • letting everything come |

It's not using one side of the brain or the other that creates chronic problems; it's *getting stuck* in one side or the other.

If muscles in and around the eyes, and the muscles of the visual reflex family, do not swing easily from relax to tense and back again, myopia, hyperopia, or strabismus will result. What you can observe on the outside is a child staring and straining to see. What is not seen is the internal imbalance and everything that implies. Slap a pair of glasses on top of that inner state and the visual, emotional dysfunction remains, even though the child may perform better in the outer world.

If the child is writing words backward, is losing his place when reading, or is unable to sit still long enough to do a vision game, the two sides of the brain may be vying for the same job. More often, one side is sulking in the closet or taking off on a rocket ship. Why? Because things may be just too hard, unpleasant, or just plain uninteresting around here.

The right brain will slam its door shut if it feels it is being criticized. The left brain will not sit down and add two and two if it thinks it's been abandoned. A child genius is using both sides of his brain. A genius is not a math whiz who cannot kick a ball. Genius does both. This is the Renaissance child with no visual blur.

# More Compassion Please

Clogged-up pathways in the brain cause a breakdown in communication, failure to perform well in school, inability to express clear feelings, and poor eyesight. This situation angers and frightens adults. Do you remember your own examples of this? "She doesn't want to hear." See if you can break the patterns of the past and find a different way to approach children, to involve them in taking care of their lives, their brain space, with laughter and enthusiasm.

To see well, both hemispheres of the brain must be switched on and working together. Certain eye and body muscles are used to glance into the distance or at the blackboard, but when we look at a picture book, those muscles must let go and let other muscles take over.

If a child is myopic, the *right brain* is switched off for the visual system. (It could still be switched on for the gross motor level, for instance, a tennis champ in glasses.)

If a child is hyperopic, the *left brain* is switched off for the visual system. (It could still be switched on for the intellectual mind, producing a stockbroker in trifocals.)

The state of affairs in the brain will generally match itself to personality and behavior patterns. Thus we find that scientific surveys match the brain scenario described above. Myopes are perfectionists, seekers after high scholastic achievement. They will often teach themselves to read, getting a head start.

Hyperopic children are clumsy by external cultural standards. To parents and teachers these cross-eyed dreamers are cloud jockeys. Sometimes the cloud is in the middle of a cyclone.

For vision improvement we wish to get the tape-recorder-brained myope to loosen up and play more. The hyperope who takes to space games anyway needs games that will merge his dancing and hyperactivity with calmly sitting still with a caterpillar: looking at small things in a relaxed fashion so he can "focus" on the words in his textbook.

## Playing in the Hemispheres

Let us explore the land of the left brain first. In this land everyone talks: they talk numbers, they talk sense. Sometimes they talk and worry. Every moment you have to decide who's right and who's wrong. All at the same time let's talk and tighten muscles. Let's talk about who's right; but more, let's talk about everything that went wrong today in detail. Do the seven-times table.

Tighten your muscles some more, including the eyes, inhale, and let go. Now we are in the right part of the brain. Do you hear that humming sound? Why, that is us! Humming, buzzing and crooning, yawning, stretching, flopping, dancing, spreading our arms, bopping. Dump all the thoughts in your head into the wastebasket and be silly.

##  Short- and Long-Term Memory Games

### For Left-Brain Training

From the cupboards and drawers find six objects that can be identified by their shape. Place the objects, without the child or children seeing them, under a towel on the table or floor. Without peeking, each child puts her hand under the towel and feels each object in turn. After taking her hand out, she tells you what the objects are. This game could be repeated at other times with different and more objects. This is left-brain training.

### For Right-Brain Training

Lie down on the floor together and palm your eyes by placing your cupped hands over your closed eyes. Take a trip back in time to your infancy. What is the first thing you remember? Talk about this. Trade memories. See if you can broaden the stage and see more items.

Another good way to activate long-term right-brain memory is to tell the child about the cute things she did as a tiny babe or little child. Here are some other springboards: "Remember your fourth birthday. What happened on that day?" "On Christmas, when we went to visit . . ."

##  Put Your Brains Together

It's time to blend the abilities of the two hemispheres. Pick an ability from the left side and combine it with something from the right side.

### Drawing and Naming

Let's draw lots of pictures of things and give them names.

### Big and Little

Draw something huge. With a stick you could draw gigantic images in the sand or dirt. Make pictures on the ground with leaves. Get those images as large as possible, then reduce them to middle size. Gather twigs or pebbles and make smaller images. Go smaller still. Seeds, tiny bits of dirt. Go smaller still. How small can we get?

Sometimes a child is stubbornly stuck in a one-sided mode. Being technically correct may have won a blue ribbon in the past. In that case whimsy and coloring outside the lines may appear dangerous. If this is occurring, the best policy is to "pace" the child. Glide alongside him for a while in the activity he has chosen. Then sneak in a laugh, a joke, or a curveball along the way. Do your best not to resist the child's resistance to immediately changing brain modes. If you do, you may get a cold shoulder.

For all eyesight problems, the whole brain must get turned on, again and again and again. One of the very best ways to instantly reconcile the dueling hemispheres, the mystics with the soldiers, is with a movement called Cross-Crawl.

## Cross-Crawl Dancing

Felicity shows you the basic Cross-Crawl.

If you move your right hand and your left foot simultaneously, both hemispheres of your brain are active. It's the same for left hand and right foot. This is the movement every human infant practices from the age of eight to twelve months by creeping. Everyone benefits from repeating the basics.

Start out on the floor. Creep under the table, between the chairs. Set some goals: roll a ball into the corner of the room and crawl over to get it. Now roll it to me. Everybody stay down at rug rat level for a time.

Move to standing. With the Left and Right Song on page 65 practice finding right and left first.

### For the Rest of Your Life

Bring your left knee up and tap it with your right hand. Bring your right knee up and tap it with your left hand. Repeat Cross-Crawling until you've had

Felicity stretching in
Cross-Crawl for
tipuana seeds

enough for now. The Cross-Crawling Song on page 65 will help you remember it later.

### Variations on the Cross-Crawl

Find objects in your visual field to Cross-Crawl toward, such as the moon, a star, a hawk, a frog, a hill, a tree, your dad, the picture on the front of your mom's shirt. Myopic children should Cross-Crawl at first toward objects up close, then with shapes that are farther away. Hyperopic children do the opposite: first Cross-Crawl toward a far-off tree, then a bush; then move to a shirt button or a flower.

Do a stretching Cross-Crawl dance with your favorite music.

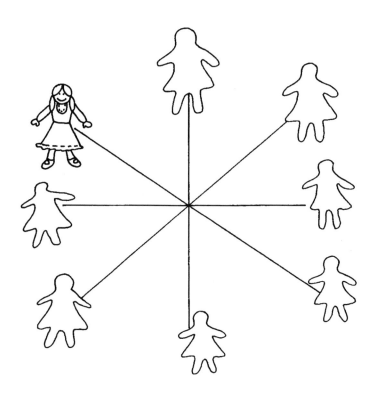

Look at me in different positions while you do your Cross-Crawl.

## LEFT AND RIGHT SONG

*Words–Traditional, Music by Elizabeth Ledger*

Put your right hand in, take your right hand out.

Now let's see if you can shake it all a-bout. Put your left hand in, take your

left hand out. That's what it's all a - bout.

Put your right foot in...
Put your right ear...
Put your right eye...
Put your right shoulder...

## CROSS-CRAWLING

*Words and Music by Elizabeth Ledger*

Cross crawl-ing, cross crawl-ing, good for my brain.

Left hand to right knee, and right hand to left knee, and do it all

o - ver a - gain.

## Timetable for Cross-Crawl

### Birth to Eight Months

This age group explores one side of the brain at a time. At four months the infant will gaze intently at an object in his two hands held right at his midline, but mostly he practices right- or left-sided movements.

### Eight to Twelve Months

Mind and body systems are ready to cross-connect the wiring. Crawling usually begins during this time. If you think your child would enjoy an integration boost, you can lay him on his back and manually touch his hand to his opposite knee.

What could interfere with the crawling practice needed to produce a brain and nervous system that will stay integrated throughout the buffets and joys of childhood?

- illness or accidents
- anxious or overambitious parents
- busy parents who keep their infants in playpens and/or walkers
- overambitious children who want to stand before they crawl
- mixed dominance (see page 68)
- the terrible baby-walker

If you see a baby-walker with a baby in it—throw a fit, for these reasons: Babies in walkers may look as if they are having fun, but they are restricted from the touching and grabbing that foster hand-eye coordination. A child's weight in an upright position puts stress on the spine at too early an age. Fifteen thousand baby-walker accidents per year are reported in the United States. Children scoot by too fast for parents to stop them from going over an edge or down the stairs. These babies don't yet have input from eyes, hands, and feet concerning empty space.

Do not despair if your child missed out on the necessary amount of crawling to reliably wire his nervous system during the eight-to-twelve-months window. It is always possible to reestablish Cross-Crawl and repair the wiring job. Crawling is used in remedial reading programs. Many chiropractors recommend this movement to their patients. It is standard practice in every Natural Vision Improvement class. An NVI student and great-grandmother, Dorothy Bryce, touches opposite hand to knee when she wants to remember where she put her keys. This works for every human, including those in wheelchairs or lying in hospital beds.

### One to Five Years

Let's be a cat and scratch fleas in Cross-Crawl fashion. Let's do Cross-Crawl while Dad holds out favorite toys at different positions: up high, down low, to the right, to the left, in the distance, and finally up close. Watch that toy move to different positions while you're Cross-Crawling, so both sides of your brain are activated no matter which direction you look. Give your toy a hug. And Dad too.

The infinity sign reminds your brain to "get it together."

### Five to Twelve Years

This is the age where children become self-contained. They engage in abstraction. Forming clubs is a natural to balance musing. Form a "Lonely Brains Club" for dance parties.

Get your crayons and lots of paper. Draw the infinity sign. This sign says "get it together" to your brain. Both hemispheres put down their weapons or get-away cars and frolic with each other like otters underwater. Put these infinity signs everywhere your eyes might fall upon them—on the fridge if you want to lose weight, on the computer, over your bed, inside a cupboard. If you have a task at school to perform, a test or math homework to do, always do Cross-Crawl and draw the infinity sign at the top of your page before beginning. (Cross-Crawl can even be done secretly under the desk or at the bus stop by making small movements with the fingers of one hand and the toes of the opposite foot, then repeating it on the other side.)

Use the Cross-Crawl movements as a stress breaker with any activity, with schoolwork, and especially in combination with all the vision-improvement games coming up. If at any time you find yourself struggling with the vision games, return to Cross-Crawl dancing.

# The Question of Dominance

Dominance really means leadership and support. A good leader in the body receives sensory input, makes a decision, and delegates execution of the decision. Human beings take input through their five senses, then act through the motor system of the body.

"Normal" dominance would have the dominant leader brain on one side and all the executive motor agents dominant on the other side. For example, Mary is right-brain dominant. If she supports herself on her left foot to kick a ball, listens with her left ear, and looks through a telescope with her left eye, then she has a normal dominance pattern. For an easy life she ought to be left-handed. Some NVI students remember being forced to use their right hand when they preferred to use their left. These people are still dealing with being punished for their natural inclinations.

"Mixed" dominance occurs when the leader brain is on one side and the ears, eyes, hands, and feet are switching sides. Xavier has a dominant left brain. He uses his right hand to write and his left foot for support, and he listens to the radio with the speaker in his left ear. No wonder his nervous system gets confused and takes its own sweet time in passing memos around. Children and adults with mixed dominance need brain integration games every day.

I have not yet found a myope or hyperope with a completely normal dominance pattern.

If you wish to find out more about dominance patterns in your family members, consult a Natural Vision Improvement teacher or Educational Kinesiology practitioner. I feel that awareness of the chaos produced by mixed dominance grants us understanding and patience with everyone's behavior.

# 8

# Eyes Must Move to See

## Eyes Grasp the World with Saccadic Motion

The essential rapid flickering of eyes is called saccadic motion. In 1964 the Russian biophysicist Alfred Yarbus demonstrated that if this motion stops, an "empty field" is created within one to three seconds. "Empty field" means no shapes, no colors; nothing is seen.

You can observe saccadic eye movements yourself. Find someone to get close to. Watch her eyeball from the side. As your specimen looks straight ahead, you will see her eye making small jerky hops. This happens even when the person thinks she is "fixing" her gaze on something.

To imagine how far your eyeball travels during an average saccadic hop, cut a pie into ten thousand pieces. Eyeballs travel across one of these pieces in one-fiftieth of a second. Then they change direction.

I call this gyrating movement of the eyeballs the saccadic dance. If the saccadic dance is slowed down, visual clarity is inhibited. Research saccadic eye movements of people who wear thick glasses (ask them to remove their specs); then observe people with normal vision. Long, languid saccades accompany refractive error compared with the sparkling agile motion of normal sight.

Everyone benefits from swinging and swaying. It is relaxing to body and mind. By using the swinging and movement games in this chapter, we invite the saccadic dance to return or to remain in everyone's eyes. The dance takes place in the context of total body aliveness. Head moves, eyelids blink, lungs inflate and deflate. The whole dance hall is pulsing to the beat, even with tranquil music.

I never use the word *focus*, either in this book or when teaching. The word *focus* is a left-brain word that connotes fixing your gaze on something. People with refractive error are already trying too hard to focus, staring and mentally working to see something. No more of that please.

Record of infant's eye movements during free examination of the photo of a human face (below) with both eyes for three minutes

Girl from Volga (photo by S. Fredlyand)

Eyes instinctively dance around shapes that give survival and social information.

Saccadic movements around a little girl's face are depicted in the top left illustration. They show how an infant's eyes would track a human face.

# Babies Don't Stare

### Observations of Aerro's Mother

At thirteen to fourteen days, Aerro begins to noticeably track objects. When he is swung back and forth he will strongly and sometimes very swiftly move his head to follow an image. He seems to follow in this manner most especially images with a strong light-and-dark contrast, such as a lightbulb or the hill line at sunset (dark hills with light coming from behind), or changing patterns of high contrast.

At sixteen days he appears to concentrate more frequently on his parents' faces. We, his parents, behave in ways to encourage these actions, by looking for images to draw his attention to and by attempting to gain his attention and making faces for him.

Day 18: Visually he is very interested in the motion of his environment. When he is in input mode (i.e., having been fed and changed, awake and looking around), he becomes bored after a few minutes of lying still by himself and begins to fuss and cry. When he is picked up and carried around, he immediately stops fussing and looks everywhere. When he is carried around the house, he swivels his head to track various images. It now becomes apparent that he directs his attention toward sources of light, especially windows and door frames.

He also enjoys lying in one's arms on his back, with his head lying back over one arm so that he is *looking at everything upside down*. So at this point he is not *recognizing*, he is purely *inputting*. He will stay in this position happily for quite a while looking around. If he is also in motion, that is, being rocked, swung, bounced on the trampoline, he will turn his head back and forth a great deal, tracking images. He also enjoys music while doing this (many kinds, from Benny Goodman to Hall and Oats to Led Zeppelin) and will often fall asleep.

*Note:* He really enjoys motion in general, and this is usually the way to calm him, whether his eyes are open or closed. A flash thought: could this have any correlation to the necessity of movement during labor for stress relief (the stress brought by pain)? For him movement is soothing of various baby stresses. All humans need to move to release energy. When we are so small that we cannot really move ourselves, it seems that rocking and moving by the parents is what allows that energy release for the infant.

## Rock-a-Bye My Baby

One of the most important items for baby raising is a rocking chair. Rocking soothes mama and calms the baby. For nursing and feeding, it is a must. If you bottle-feed, please alternate holding the infant on right and left sides. This ensures that each eye gets stimulation during the pleasant act of suckling.

## Rocking, Rolling, Bouncing

### A Voice to the Child

"Inside your mama's uterus you were constantly tumbled and vibrated. Maybe your mother went for long walks; perhaps she danced or made love. Her heart was pumping close to your ears. You were born in movement and rhythms. Your caregivers instinctively pat and jounce you when you're hollering. Maybe they want some peace and quiet. It usually works. Rocking you in a chair will entertain your eyes and brain with gently moving shapes. Some babies' caregivers bought a minitrampoline and found that you love the tiny bounces that the two of you can make on it. It puts you to sleep when you get too heavy to hold, and it pumps the lymph fluid between all the cells in your body."

Bounce your baby to sleep.

A minitrampoline is a tool to use all one's life. It keeps people healthy and fit without jogging on a hard road. It is a lifesaver for people sitting all day in front of a computer as I am right now. The minitramp is two meters (six feet) away from me, flat on the floor—not propped against a wall, or hidden in the closet. Children make a beeline for it at Vision Playcamps.

Lymphatic pumping is good for what ails anyone. Blood is moved through the human body by the heart. Your heart will do its job even when you spend a year lying on your back. Not so the lymph system, which sweeps away waste products from cells. The lymphatic network operates like canals with locks. Only movement of legs and arms opens and closes the lock. Walking while swinging your arms in Cross-Crawl fashion releases lymph locks and keeps this fluid moving. So does gentle bouncing on a well-made

Bouncing upward closes lymph locks. Falling downward opens lymph locks.

minitrampoline. I say "gentle" because too many folks think they have to start out with hard jumping. This aggravates the bladder, which first needs conditioning. Please start out on the trampoline with tiny bounces for only three minutes. You can build up from there. Hold your baby in your arms to joggle him to sleep. Aerro's favorite music for this was nuns singing Gregorian chants. When he was too big to hold, he lay on a blanket between my legs on the minitramp. At the top of the bounce you and baby are weightless, gravity-free for a split second.

Astronauts reported seeing trucks on highways from their perch in outer space. This superhuman acuity of vision could be attributed to weightlessness. There is no gravity drag on the eye muscles, therefore saccadic motion is faster.

Janet and vision teachers swinging triplets

## Dance of the Eaglet Swing

Hold baby facing outward. Turn your whole body from side to side in half a circle. Keep your shoulders aligned with your hips. This turning is done totally by your feet like a golfer's swing. Your left heel goes out as your weight shifts to your right foot. Your right foot swings out away from you as your weight shifts to your left foot. You cannot see the child's face, but be assured she is checking out all available visual shapes. This swing can also be done in front of a mirror. You and baby can check each other out as your images swing past.

## Faces

Babies are interested in other humans, especially the eyes, noses, and mouths of those bigger creatures who are constantly peering into their cribs. Newborns will spend their leisure time cooing at abstract human faces. Place an image like the one at left in your baby's view at a distance of approximately twenty-two centimeters (seven to ten inches). The image should be enlarged on a photocopier to be ten centimeters wide (four inches). This prepares her for relating to the new faces that will come later. Use the image from this page and/or cut out models from magazines. Spend time with your infant face-to-face. Notice how she examines you and her brothers and sisters peacefully. Watch for the saccadic dance of her eyes on your moving lips and eyes.

You could use animal faces also. Yarbus's research shows that human eyes saccadically trace animal faces just as they do human faces.

##  Make a Mobile

Eyes are attracted to edges and motion. Anything that sparkles, moves, glitters, reflects light, will entertain your child's innate desire to see the world in action. Homemade mobiles can be put together in your kitchen. A newborn won't pull them into her mouth until she is about four months old. At first, place them within the twenty-two centimeters (seven to eight inches) range. Later you will have to move mobiles out of reach unless they are chewable.

You will need coat hangers and some string or yarn. Gather household objects such as key rings, feathers, playing cards, cereal boxes, plastic measuring spoons, kitchen sponges, costume jewelry. Attach them to the coat hangers. Enlarge the shapes at right on a photocopier or draw them with black paint or crayon. Paste them onto cardboard and attach them to the mobile.

### Babies Want to Kick and Bat

Move all visual mobiles out of reach and replace them with mobiles made of soft lightweight objects that can be kicked and pulled. Paint black lines and dots on Ping-Pong balls with indelible markers or crayons. Make two slits in the balls and hang them from the "bat mobile"; you can also add rag dolls, ribbons, plastic streamers. Take some wide elastic from the sewing basket; tie it tightly across the crib. Attach a plastic bottle, a measuring cup, and a wooden spoon with more wide elastic.

# Muscles behind the Movement

Six husky eye muscles move eyeballs around. Like every other muscle in the body, eye muscles take their directives from the brain. Our desire is to *keep the eye muscles relaxed and flexible* through movement games, not to make them work harder.

The right brain tells muscles to relax and lengthen. The left brain tells muscles to tighten up and shorten. Proper muscle response needs both actions and both sides of the brain. The muscles moving the eyeballs work in pairs—one must pull while the other lets go. One partner pulling all the time will produce a turned eye. Two partners pulling all the time could produce hyperopia. Oblique muscles wrapped too tightly around the eyeball could create an elongated myopic eyeball. (*Note:* This is not a popular theory with the optical industry.)

Muscles of the left eye

1   **Superior rectus turns the eye upward and inward.**
2   **Superior oblique turns the eye downward and outward.**
3   **Sphenoid bone.**
4   **Medial rectus turns eye inward.**
5   **Lateral rectus turns eye outward.**
6   **Inferior rectus turns eye downward and inward.**
7   **Inferior oblique turns eye upward and outward.**

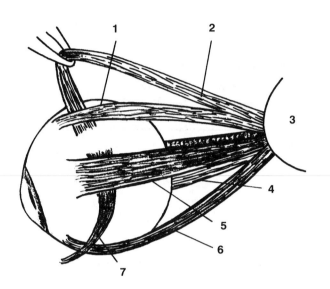

## Eye Muscles

Imagine what would occur if one partner were switched off, deactivated. The other partner would have to do the whole dance by herself. She tries mighty hard but cannot win the dance marathon alone. Eventually she collapses. "Help! We need stronger glasses." The secret is not what most people think: "to work at focusing." This results in even more stress, fatigue, and blur. The stare takes over. Anyone with functional visual blur (as opposed to blur caused by disease or accident) engages in expert staring. It's the glassy look on the lonesome dancer's face.

# How We Create Blurred Vision

"The cause of all imperfect sight is staring," wrote Dr. William Bates. What's a stare? It's the opposite of an easy, soft, alive saccadic dance. This is why we have encouraged babies' eyes to stay loose with mobiles and the Dance of the Eaglet.

Staring becomes an unconscious body-mind habit. Changing the habit of staring helps vision improve. But first let's get a hold on staring in every way we can.

## Play a Staring Game

Everyone produce a good hard stare; a mad stare; a sad stare. If you have normal vision, notice how much energy it takes to hold a stare. Notice that it's close to impossible for you to stare for very long. While struggling to hold a fixed stare, you may become aware of the saccadic motion of your eyes. If you do wear glasses, notice how easy it is for you to stare. It's an old habit, diligently practiced. To make a really good stare you have to park your eyes somewhere, tighten your jaw, stiffen shoulders and neck, tighten your tummy, and hold your breath. If you can manage to worry about something, that helps tremendously with staring. Feel the stare all over your body; be aware of how much energy it uses up. Now do the opposite: Breathe. Let your shoulders *d-o-w-n-n-n*. Massage them. Massage your neck. Yawn a big yawn and find your Magic Nose Pencil.

Flynn staring

##  The Magic Nose Pencil

It may be hiding in your pocket, or in the back of your shirt, or it could be sitting on top of your ear. Here's what the Magic Pencil looks like. Its true home is on the end of your nose.

The Magic Nose Pencil, alias the Magic Pencil, is our most important tool for breaking the stare and establishing or reestablishing a good habit of saccadic movement. This makes lots of "nose penciling," edging, and tracing necessary for both myopes and hyperopes.

Draw everything with your Magic Nose Pencil, moving your head slightly. Eyes *automatically* seek the edges of shapes, too fast to think about it. If you hold your head still, only moving your eyeballs, you gum up the vision works. Move your whole head as you sketch with your pencil. Be more like a gesticulating Italian than a proper British professor. Relatively few Italians wear glasses. They just make gorgeous frames.

Let's do some drawing and coloring to get used to the Magic Nose Pencil idea. Dick Bruna's picture books for children have been praised for their simple line drawings. Edged in solid black, a little girl in bright red feeds black-edged buns to well-defined ducks.

Make your own pictures in this style on paper. Use a thick black crayon for drawing the shapes. Then fill in those shapes with brilliant colors. As you draw, keep your Magic Nose Pencil moving loosely along with the motion of your hands. When you've drawn enough Bruna-style pictures, put crayons and paper aside.

Put a pencil up to your nose. Imagine it gets long enough to reach to your dad. Put a pretend black line around him. Do it with your sister, then with the cat.

Start drawing the furniture. Drop the physical pencil, but pretend it is still there on the end of your nose. It can telescope. It gets long when you are drawing something in the distance. It shortens when you sketch something up close. Go outside with your Magic Nose Pencil, which is, of course, invisible. Draw everything around you, one shape at a time. You never have to finish a drawing, nor do you have to be careful about fine details. Loose, even sloppy drawing and edging is better than trying to be too careful about detail. The song below will help you remember to edge with the Magic Nose Pencil in

**MAGIC PENCIL**

*Music – Traditional, Words by Janet Goodrich*

Mag-ic Pen-cil, Mag-ic Pen-cil, I love you, I love you.

All a-round the kit-chen, All a-round the kit-chen, I draw you,

I draw you.

All around the classroom
All around the highway
All around my bedroom
All around the garden

All around the music
All around my family
All around the people
All around the foodstore

**Make up any more you like!**

school, in the car, at the computer. When you talk with a friend, draw her face: eyes and nose and mouth, plus earrings and gold chains.

## Trace It

Place a picture flat against a window so that daylight shines through it. Place a sheet of plain paper over it and trace the image you want with a pen. Do lots of tracing. Then leave the pieces of paper behind. Go outside to a hillside or a patio. Pretend your tracing pencil is on the end of your nose. How many shapes can you find? Tiny green bugs, flowers, cars, your toys and stuffed animals. Line them all up and trace their shapes.

## TV Eyes

Parents are worried about the hours their children spend glued to the TV. I would be too. American children spend an average of six hours a day in front of the TV. Staring into a TV set keeps their eyes fixed at one distance. It disallows near-and-far practice. Hands sit idle and imagination is canned. However, if the demand for TV watching is overwhelming, consider using it as a vision training tool. When my children were small, we rented a TV set each year for the month of December. You can make good use of TV for this short period: turn watching Christmas cartoons into a vision game. Trace the edges of the cartoons on the screen with your Magic Nose Pencils.

## Frogs on Lily Pads

Scatter several bath towels on the floor. These are lily pads. Sit on your lily pad and croak like a frog for a while, sketching the world around you with your Magic Nose Pencil. Crawl or hop to the next lily pad. Sketch the world again. If you have different-colored towels you could match the color of your Magic Nose Pencil to that of each towel. Pink towel: pink Nose Pencil. Sketch all the pink objects in your visual world.

## Take Your Magic Nose Pencil through the Maze

Take a piece of paper and make your own maze. Trace through the maze with your Magic Nose Pencil.

## Join the Dots

Make your own join-the-dots game—join the dots with a real pencil, then with your Magic Nose Pencil.

##  The Magic Nose Paintbrush

Everyone sit down comfortably. Imagine you have a Magic Paintbrush on the end of your nose.

It gets shorter when you paint things up close and longer when you paint things in the distance. Whatever color you imagine in your mind will automatically come flowing out the end of your Magic Nose Paintbrush. With your eyes closed, paint a red apple sitting on your hand. Feel the weight of the apple. Take a bite out of the apple. How does it taste?

Now let's paint a giant apple in the sky, a huge red spaceship-sized apple. Cover every bit of the apple spaceship with sticky red paint. This could take a while. Where does the spaceship go when you finish painting it? Paint other objects that become real.

## Painting Pictures Game

Painting pictures in your mind uses all parts of your brain. In addition the movement of your swishing brush produces saccadic motion.

Start with a picture from a favorite book held at a comfortable distance. Scan across the picture, soaking in the details. (Many picture books lend themselves well to Painting Pictures. Alison Lester's book *Imagine* gives planetary settings from the Arctic to the jungle. When you get really good at painting pictures, you can advance to complex images such as those in *The Boy Who Painted the Sun* by Jill Morris or *Animalia* by Graeme Base.) After three minutes of scanning, close your eyes. You become a master at scene painting. Use the picture-book images as your take-off point. Close your eyes; with a Magic Paintbrush on your nose that squirts out exactly the color you imagine, lavishly paint shapes, settings, characters for five to ten minutes.

Blink open your eyes, scan the same picture again, exclaiming how much brighter, three-dimensional, sharper, and real it has become. You can do this procedure several times in a row with the same picture.

This game is endless and can be used anywhere, anytime. The painting motion keeps neck and eye muscles loose as a goose. Right-brain imagination is stimulated. Painting Pictures relaxes us all. It produces creative, fun people with Technicolor, internal traveling theaters.

## Bird Swing

Do the Bird Swing outdoors or indoors with music. Tune in to your birdness. Standing with your feet firmly on the ground, swing your body in half a circle with or without baby brother. The fluffy, fantastic, flexible, telescoping Magic Feather on the end of your nose swings with you, tickling everything in sight. And everything out of sight.

When grass gets tickled, it giggles. When trees get tickled they sigh with pleasure. When Dad gets tickled he grins. When the dog gets tickled with the

Kylie and Aerro do the Bird Swing together.

Magic Nose Feather, she howls. Everything responds when touched by your Magic Feather, which sits on the end of your nose.

You can also tickle things secretly with your Magic Nose Feather: people in the street, the carrot in your hand just before you crunch into it. Everything comes alive when brushed with your Magic Nose Feather. As you are tickling the world with your Magic Nose Feather, you could sing the song below.

# I WILL TICKLE WHAT I SEE

*Music – Traditional, Words by Janet Goodrich*

I will tic-kle what I see,   what I see, what I see.   I will tic-kle what I see,

With my ru - by feath - er.

2. With my bright orange feather.
3. With my yellow feather.
4. With my emerald feather.
5. With my light green feather.
6. With my sapphire feather.
7. With my indigo feather.
8. With my violet feather.

## 👁 The Near-Far Swing

The Near-Far Swing is good for both myopes and hyperopes. It helps myopes bring their clear close vision outward into the distance, just like unrolling a royal carpet. Hyperopes can bring their relaxed distance vision in close with this swing.

Sit comfortably indoors or outside and find an object to hold in your hand. This could be a toy, a blade of grass, your watch. Choose an object in the distance anywhere from one meter (three feet) away to the horizon. A tree will do or a license plate on a car or a picture on the wall.

Fiona doing the Near-Far Swing with a sunflower up close and a tree in the distance

Connect your close object and your far object with an invisible rope. Circle the close object a few times with your nose, then slide and glide on the rope out to your distant object. Don't slide near and far with your eyeballs. Move your head, letting your nose guide your eyes.

Circle your distant object a few times, then slide back on the rope to the object in your hand. This is a Near-Far Swing. Your rope could turn into a string of pearls, a spider's thread, a gold chain. Repeat the Near-Far Swing at least ten times on the same object, then choose another two shapes: one up close, the other in the distance.

The Near-Far Swing is fun in the house, in the kitchen, at the table. It's intriguing on a mountaintop. You could create invisible lines of force making a network across the countryside.

**I CAN LOOK**

*Words and Music by Donald Woodward*

I can look ve-ry near, I can look ve-ry close,
I can look ve-ry far, gaze up to all the stars, Or

Cir-cl-ing what I see be-fore_____ me,_____
o-ver the dis-tant hor-i_____ zon._____

I can look ve-ry near, I can look ve-ry close, And
I can look ve-ry far, gaze up to all the stars, And

I will see what I want to see._____
I will see what I want to see._____

## Ball Games Galore

Balls are attractive to eyes. Their roundness, unpredictability, and free-flowing movement irresistibly beckon interest and induce saccadic motion. Nothing moves as superbly as a ball—except perhaps the human eyeball itself. Cultivate all ball games to call forth flickery, faster-than-you-can-think-about-it saccadic eye movements. Buy your family a collection of balls big and little, spongy ones and bouncy ones. Have a special box or basket to keep them in.

- Roll the ball. Follow the ball with your nose.
- Bounce the ball. Follow the ball with your nose
- Play catch. Follow the ball with your nose.

**ROLL THE BALL**

*Words and Music by Donald Woodward*

Add in anybody's name to sing and play this game with - Mommy, Michael, Katie, Jimmy, Grandma, Chinta - whoever!!

## The Rainbow Ribbon Wand

Make everyone a Rainbow Ribbon Wand. It brings together switching on the whole brain, movement, rhythm, total body and eye coordination. Attach a 16-millimeter-wide ribbon (about 1/2 inch wide) that is 2 meters (about 2 yards) long to a piece of dowel. The dowel could be 16 to18 millimeters (about 1/2 inch) in diameter. The length of this stick should be about 52.4 centimeters (20 5/8 inches) long. (This length is the Egyptian cubit, a unit of measure that is meant to give strength to the body.) Fasten the ribbon to the end of the stick with a thumbtack. A lovely "lazy eight" infinity sign pattern can now be made with the Rainbow Ribbon Wand. Turn on some music, sing, or hum while making lovely patterns in the air with your Rainbow Ribbon Wand. Follow its pattern with your nose and feel yourself getting switched on.

Eleanor making an infinity sign with her Rainbow Ribbon Wand

## Blinking

After every blink, your retina ships millions of bits of new data along the optic nerve cable to your brain. Blinking briefly turns off all entering light, giving retinal cells a short rest in the darkness. Then eyelids lift and a whole new light show is presented. Blinking also contributes to the constant vibration of living eyes. If you were inside your eyeball, a blink would feel like a Richter-eight earthquake.

The frame of a TV picture flashes past in 0.033 seconds. A blink takes only 0.025 seconds. Most people blink an average of twenty times per minute. They blink less when they are angry or anxious or when they need to stay alert. A constant internal state of left-brain tension causes some people to hold their eyelids up until visual fatigue sets in. Then a slow effortful blink is made. These people especially need blinking practice to relax their eyelid muscles and their nerves. A bit of deep breathing and blinking helps clear everyone's vision. You can practice happy blinking with our two blinking songs.

### THE BLINKING SONG

*Music – Traditional, Words by NVI Teacher Dede Callichy*

Blink, blink, blink your eyes, Gent - ly blink your eyes.

Lu - bri - cate and cleanse and rest, Gent - ly blink your eyes.

## KIBATLA, OUBONA* SIROUROU BELL

*Music – Traditional South African Song, Words by NVI Teacher Dede Callichy*

**With a Swing**

I want to see a but-ter-fly blink, Ki-

bat- la, ou-bo-na-*, si- rou-rou- bell.

\* - indicates to blink, click fingers and tongue, all at the same time!

I want to see a crocodile blink, kibatla, oubona * sirourou bell.
I want to see an elephant blink, kibatla, oubona * sirourou bell.
I want to see a rhinoceros blink, kibatla, oubona * sirourou bell.

Continue changing animals.

## IT'S COOL TO BE A LION

*Words and Music by Bernard O'Scanaill*

**Slowly, In Two**

It's cool to be a li - on, just stretch-ing in the sun.    I

stretch all day, from break-fast time, 'til it's near-ly half past one.

It's cool to be a lion,
And a lazy lion too.
I yawn all day from breakfast time,
'Til it's nearly half past two.

It's cool to be a lion,
Just swinging in a tree.
I swing all day from breakfast time,
'Til it's nearly half past three.

It's cool to be a lion,
I breathe deep when I roar.
I roar and breathe from breakfast time,
'Til it's nearly half past four.

##  Breathing and Yawning

Eyes and brains need lots of oxygen. Deep breathing, sighing with a sound, and noisy yawning provide humans, lions, tigers, hippos, and lots of other creatures with necessary oxygen. Yawning also releases muscles reflexive to the visual system—trapezius and neck flexors. It softens facial muscles and helps you change your state of mind. Your eyes give themselves a bath by yawning. Vision brightens up as if you had washed the world as well as your eyes. Make a sound with your exhalation. This could be a loud roar with the lions. At the very least give a gentle sigh.

## Swing It, Sing It, Dance It

Make movement games part of your family lifestyle. Adult vision will improve also. More help for adults in glasses can be obtained through the Natural Vision Improvement book. My cassette tapes are great for using in a portable cassette player while walking or driving. Sing eye songs while walking to school, at the dinner table, in the bath.

---

## Timetable for Movement

### Birth to One Year +

Set up mobiles. Swing, rock, and gently bounce babies until they are just too heavy to hold.

### One to Five Years +

This is the time for dancing, looking near and far, and ball games galore. Blink, stretch, yawn.

### Five to Twelve Years +

Introduce the Magic Nose Pencil, Feather, and Paintbrush. Do the Near-Far Swing, Yawning, and Painting Pictures game. Make everyone a Rainbow Ribbon Wand.

---

# Nuclear Vision

Your mind, eyes, and brain have a common characteristic. They use the concepts of foreground and background in the same way a landscape artist does. However, a painting on the wall is flat and static. The paintings created in our visual system are dimensional and constantly in flux.

Interest determines foreground. One day while crossing the street in Los Angeles, I was nearly hit by a car. I distinctly remember a series of sharp colored images—a shiny fender, a red panel, a black glob of tar suddenly in the foreground. The sky, buildings, and trees were in that moment dulled in color and blurred. They became background. My feet pushed me away from the car without consulting my left brain. I thumped on the car and yelled, "Are you blind?" The driver wasn't blind; he just wasn't interested in pedestrians. "Sorry, I didn't see you." It was a good thing I had not been staring. I avoided injury because important bits of light were fed into my fovea centralis and visual brain in a hundredth of a second. And the memo reached my feet in time.

Quickness of eye, mind, and brain is slowed down by all the stress factors that interfere with brain integration and with the passage of messages from

"Sharpshooter" eyesight comes from the fovea centralis.

1  Optic nerve
2  Blood vessels
3  Retina
4  Lens
5  Ciliary muscle
6  Iris
7  Pupil
8  Cornea
9  Fovea centralis, "Conedominium"
10  Macula lutea, "Cone Village"

one hemisphere to the other and to the hands and feet. If the light beams from that front fender had not entered my fovea I could be limping today. If I had been in a myopic stare, or worrying about being hit by a car, the lightning-rapid foveal messages could have been delayed.

People with refractive error have lowered foveal or central vision. My name for this ability to see clearly what you are interested in is Nuclear Vision. This "sharpshooter" eyesight can be recovered and honed with Nuclear Vision games. Nuclear Vision is *not concentration and a tight focus*, where all peripheral shapes are blanked out. Sharp central vision needs peripheral, background blur for its very existence. It is a paradox. If a person with refractive error fights the blur and tries harder to see, she will create more blur. Clarity needs blur just as the distinct foreground of a painting needs a hazy background, just as day needs night. Surprisingly, heightening the blur makes sharp central vision reappear. The following Nuclear Vision games will help everyone restore excellent central vision.

## A Trip to Fovea Centralis

Everyone lie down and close your eyes. Let's hop into a boat and blow magic shrinkage dust over it. It gets smaller and smaller. It gets so small we can float right through the pupil of our eye, through the lens of our eye, back to a spreading, curved, red wall called the retina.

Notice the rich orange color of this healthy retina. See crimson red rivers ladened with oxygen-rich blood. These streams feed our cone and rod cells with nutrients. Larger blue rivers are carrying garbage away from the cells. Out here in the countryside (the outer areas of our retina), rods that see black and white and cones that see color and details live side by side. This is blur country. Everyone here is laid-back and not too hyped up about making things clear. In fact our rod cells still use old-fashioned party-line phones— six to a line. As you know, all the phone lines from retinal nerve cells end up in the brain. At night our brain gets very unclear and vague messages about the shapes out in that big space on the other side of our pupil.

Now I want to show you our greatest pride and joy. If you will kindly take a direct line from the center of your pupil right back to the center of your retina, you will find, I am proud to announce, a village that was built here many years ago. It's called Cone Village. Some folks who dig Latin call it the macula lutea. Only cones are allowed to reside in Cone Village. No whites or blacks allowed: only colors. Every single cone cell in that village

# WHEN I COUNT

*Words by Janet Goodrich, Music by Donald Woodward*

When I count I cir-cle a-round and a-round, a-round and a-round, a-round and a-round. When I count I cir-cle a-round and a-round, with my Mag-ic Fea-ther. I am count-ing flow-ers and beans, flow-ers and beans, flow-ers and beans. I am count-ing flow-ers and beans, with my Mag-ic Fea-ther. One flow-er, two flow-ers, three flow-ers, four. One bean, two beans, three beans, four. When I

NOTE: This last counting section gets longer for each verse. After the last verse, return to the beginning, then finish at *Fine*

I am counting leaves on the trees, leaves on the trees, leaves on the trees...
One leaf, two leaves, three leaves, four leaves, five.
When I count I circle around...

I am counting bees and birds, bees and birds, bees and birds...
One bee, two bees, three bees, four bees, five bees, six.
One bird, two birds, three birds, four birds, five birds, six birds, seven.
When I count I circle around...

I am counting clouds in the sky, cars on the road, clouds in the sky...
One cloud, two clouds, three clouds, four clouds, five clouds, six clouds, seven clouds, eight.
One car, two cars, three cars, four cars, five cars, six cars, seven cars, eight cars, nine cars, ten!
When I count I circle around...

has its own phone. The phones are red, blue, and green. Now take a look at that high-rise inside Cone Village. That's the Conedominium. Our Latin visitors call it fovea centralis. You can see how cone cells are packed in there bottom to bottom. There are twelve million of them living in that small area. When you get a flash of crystal-clear vision, the cone phones in the Conedominium are ringing something fierce. Your color and detail vision go right over the moon.

If you would like to invest more time in the thrills and ecstasy of Nuclear Vision, play the following games. Nuclear Vision games will sharpen your already brilliant mind, help you conquer schoolwork, and get your arrow right in the bull's-eye.

## Intensify the Blur

It's strange. The way to clear vision is not to try to see your object of interest more clearly but to intensify the blurry surroundings. You do this by talking to them. When you are circling a red petunia, ask all the other flowers to be less bright, less alive than your petunia. Corbett teachers had children do this with two candles. Hold two lighted candles about twenty-six centimeters (one foot) apart. Swing your attention from one candle to the other. Pause at one candle and tell the other candle to be blurred. Keep on doing this as you gradually bring the two candles together. Penlights or colored pencils work just as well as candles.

## The Nuclear Junk Box

Fill a box with all kinds of things: bottle tops, feathers, keys, marbles, screws, pet pebbles. Dump the contents out on the table, floor, or ground. Circle each item with your nose, thereby moving your whole head. That's your foreground object. Tell all the other pieces of junk to "blur off." They constitute your background. Emphasize the blurriness of the background. You'll notice the object of your attention becomes clearer.

## Counting games

There are zillions of seashells strewn on the beach. When you start to count them, you have to single out one seashell at a time. The light beams reflected off the mass of seashells is the background. The shell you assign a numeral to is, in that moment, your foreground. Its light beams ought to ring the phones in your Conedominiums. On the beach you would do this by circling individual seashells with your nose and crying out, "One seashell," then "Two seashells," "Three seashells." Continue to count as high as you would like, always circling and being aware that the other seashells are more blurred than the one you are circling. How many different objects can you count in this way? Do your counting with a song (page 90). It's music for your right brain and numbers for your left brain.

## Hidden Pictures

Hidden Pictures games hone your ability to keep one shape constant in your mental and visual foreground, even as you move through a varied background (which could be a jungle where only the sharp-eyed stay relaxed and alive). On the opposite page, Con the Caveman is looking for his lost pets. Help him find them. This game requires at least two players. The Finder Player closes her eyes while the Describing Player picks out an animal from the picture and gives its name to the Finder. The Finder paints this animal with her Magic Nose Paintbrush for a few seconds.

The Finder opens her eyes while retaining the image of the animal in the back of her mind. The Finder scans the prehistoric landscape with a Magic Nose Feather until the creature imagined comes alive and leaps out of the background. The Finder must then celebrate in an appropriate manner to the applause of the Describer. I'm so much more interested in the process of this game than whether you get the right answer that I don't even give you the answers in the back of this book.

## Nuclear Vision on Eye Charts

Put an eye chart on the wall where you can see the top three rows on the chart clearly (page 129). Circle one letter and tell all the other letters to blur off. Move to another letter or shape and tell all the other shapes to blur off. Notice that the shape you are circling gets clearer, all by itself.

## Timetable for Nuclear Vision Games

### Birth to Five Years

During this period a natural interchange of sounds, songs, words, and spontaneous play pave the way to Nuclear Vision.

### Five to Twelve Years +

By this age the concept of "blurring off" peripheral shapes can be introduced. Use candles and junk box activities to get the idea and feeling of Nuclear Vision. Then use your Magic Nose Paintbrushes to circle and count shapes in picture books and on eye charts. It's fair to use Nuclear Vision when taking eye tests.

# 9

# Mad about Sunlight

## Are Sunglasses Good for Kids?

It had been raining in Germany for ten days. When the gray drizzle finally stopped, I stood on the veranda of the seminar house and welcomed the sun as it peeked over the lofty oak trees. Diamond droplets glittered on every leaf. I closed my eyes, drinking in warm, cleansing sunlight. I was alone that morning on the veranda until a participant in a yoga course walked past. "Beautiful!" she exclaimed as she noticed how much I was enjoying the morning glow. As she exited the veranda she turned and shot back at me, "But the sun is dangerous."

When I mention that Germans who speak English can take the instructor's course in Australia, their eyes glaze over with fear. "But what about the hole in the ozone right above Australia?" they ask. Australian government campaigns convince people they must slap on sunscreen and pop on sunglasses as soon as they step out the door. Many parents buy infant sunglasses and tie them on the baby's head. There is a rumor that sunglasses may become part of required school uniforms in schools in Brisbane.

UV anxiety sells shiploads of Taiwanese sunglasses and tons of chemical soups for the skin. The general public rarely hears about the beneficial aspects of UV (ultraviolet) light. It is true that too much UV light can burn the skin and the eyes. Too much water, heat, or vitamin A can also be harmful. There is another side to the story. Take notice when media reports and scientific irrationality overwhelm your intuition and inquiring nature. Here is what John Ott, author of *Health and Light*, says about UV light and life on planet Earth:

Another school of thought believes that while too much ultraviolet is definitely harmful, normal amounts of these forms of energy found in nature may be essential to the healthy growth and development of both plants and animals. In addition to all the new products designed to protect people from the so-called harmful effects of any trace amount of ultraviolet, come others that are designed to let through the natural ultraviolet in sunlight and add the normal amount of ultraviolet that is lacking in artificial light sources.

At Saint Paul's Catholic School in Brisbane the Bolle Company supplied free sunglasses to primary-grade children in a behavior-modification experiment to convince children to wear sunglasses all the time. Australian ophthalmologists believe that exposure to UV light causes *cataracts* (deposit of opaque substance in the lens of the eye) and *pterygiums* (a fatty yellow tissue growth on the cornea). If, they reason, children can be persuaded to wear sunglasses all their lives, when they are sixty they will not have cataracts and pterygiums. On the phone one medical expert told me his evidence was not conclusive. He is unable to do the forty- or fifty-year follow-up study that would prove that lifelong use of sunglasses will prevent eye disease, but "It's enough." When I questioned him about the research showing that some UV stimulation is essential to general health, he replied, "I'm not convinced that UV light through the eyes is important."

Other ophthalmologists believe cataracts and pterygiums are caused by faulty nutrition. Dr. Gary Price Todd states that eye diseases can be prevented and healed with nutritional supplementation.

For every scientific paper printed in ophthalmological journals there exist opposing studies by prestigious institutes denying the connection between UV light and cataracts, pterygiums, and skin cancer. On the other hand, evidence exists that humans need some UV light both on the skin to produce vitamin D and through the eyes to regulate health and happiness. Putting infants and children into sunglasses to prevent senile cataracts and pterygiums may actually have harmful side effects now.

## Light Food for Thought

Sunlight is a natural antibiotic; it destroys certain bacteria, fungi, and viruses. It prevents and heals jaundice, the inability of immature livers to detoxify bilirubin, a yellow pigment produced by dying red blood cells. The sensible thing to do with babies with jaundice would be to put them in sunlight for short periods. Babies born in hospitals spend their first few days in windowless nurseries. Those who develop jaundice are blindfolded and placed under blue fluorescent lights, a costly procedure. Giving newborns a bit of sunlight was the original cure for jaundice, and could also prevent it.

Humans are diurnal creatures. Humans are awake during the day and asleep at night, unlike the more nocturnal kangaroos and echidnas that party around my garden at night. This means that people's mental, emotional, and physical rhythms are attuned to daily sunlight.

UV light, or lack of it, affects hormone cycles. Nurses who work night shifts and sleep during the day find that their periods become abnormal and irregular. Children who attend school in buildings without windows, under fluorescent lights, show more sexual aberrations than those in rooms with windows. In Germany an architect designed a home for the blind without windows. The structure had to be promptly rebuilt. The inhabitants were getting ill from light starvation.

Sunlight on skin is necessary for vitamin D production. By 1900 the industrial cities of the world were covered by a thick blanket of smoke. Ninety percent of the children in those cities suffered from rickets; their bones were soft and deformed. Make sure your children get some sunlight on their bodies—and please don't oversoap them. Natural vitamin D is formed by the interaction of UV light with oils produced on the skin's surface. Washing with soap removes this oil. Is that why some children hate to wash? The artificial vitamin D added to milk does not have the same chemical structure as the vitamin D made by skin and UV light.

Stimulation of the endocrine system (pineal, pituitary, thyroid, parathyroid, pancreas, spleen, adrenals, and gonads), which rules growth in children, sexual behavior, appetite, mood, temperature, and metabolism, occurs through the retina of the eye. Therefore some optometrists recommend glasses that *do not* block UV light into the eyes.

Zane Kime, M.D., author of *Sunlight Can Save Your Life,* feels that UV light in the proper amount is essential for prevention of skin cancer. Wearing sunglasses may prevent your skin from getting the message to produce protective *melanin*—a preventer of skin cancer. Kime recommends gradual and moderate tanning of the skin. The only agreement is that no one should ever sunburn their skin or their eyes. Cancer cells love to multiply in an anaerobic environment. Scar tissue from long-past sunburns provides such a low-oxygen medium.

You can make sure your children do not get sunburned by covering them with clothing when they are outdoors. Kime recommends *not* using sunblocks. Slathering oils and preservatives on the skin smothers breathing pores and lends a false illusion of safety on the beach. A new sunblock has entered the market that is described as "nonchemical." Titanium dioxide flecks in this product reflect the UV light like tiny mirrors. It sounds superior to chemical UV absorbers. However, after short and sensible exposure of skin, it may be far better to cover up with clothing, wear a hat, and find the trees.

The National Council for Prevention of Cancer in the United States recommends that people not use sunglasses or sunblock. An odd possibility rears its amazing head. Could it be that the current medical and government policy of recommending sunblocks and wearing sunglasses may itself be contributing to the incidence of skin cancer?

## Why Eyes Need Sunlight

Retinal nerve cells respond only to light. Light is their food. Fish in caves and burros in mines become blind from lack of light. You certainly won't go blind from using sunglasses, but have you noticed loss of light tolerance? In 1967 I traveled to the Caribbean sporting prescription sunglasses. In the night someone sat on my backpack, smashing my glasses. The next morning I was stunned and incapacitated by the glare off sand and water. Since that time I have never worn sunglasses, not even to drive into the setting sun on Los Angeles freeways surrounded by twelve lanes of shiny clean cars. I sun my eyes in small doses at every opportunity. If you do Sunning each day for two weeks, you may no longer be bothered by glare, nor will you be squinting in the light.

After Sunning, vision is clearer and details are brighter. Kindly realize that Sunning does not mean staring with open eyes directly into the sun, as many eye professionals falsely assume. Sunning consists of closing your eyes and with relaxation moving your head around, circling the sun for ten minutes or less. You take in no more UV light than you would walking down the street or hanging clothes on the line.

The benefit is tremendous. A daily dose of UV light is supplied. The sun's warmth relaxes tight eye muscles. Retinal cells are stimulated, glare is reduced, and dispositions turn . . . sunny.

Alexandra and NVI teacher Isabele Steiner (Switzerland) sunning

### 👁 Sunning Games

Sit or stand comfortably facing the sun. Morning or afternoon is best, not high noon when the sun is directly overhead. If the sun is too bright, do your Sunning in a shady area.

Close your eyes and pretend the sun is a huge sunflower. Put a Magic Nose Feather on the end of your nose. With your Magic Feather make a circle on top of the sunflower petals. Rotate your whole head slowly, gently. Whisper "thank you" to the sun for its free gift of warmth and light and life upon the earth. Occasionally change the color of your Magic Nose Feather and sunflower to sun-kissed orange, to cherry red, to sapphire blue.

A sunflower

## Make a Sun Sandwich

After Sunning for a minute, Palm your eyes (page 106) and watch the brilliant light show that appears as afterimages dissolve from orange to red to magenta. When the light show finally slows to deep black, Sun again for a minute. Repeat the Palming. Colors will become more dramatic and your black will go velvety, like a black panther.

SUNNING SONG

*Words and Music by Bernard O'Scanaill*

With my head held high in the morn-ing sun, I feel the sun-shine tic-kle my nose. And it feels all soft and tic-kl-y, Like a ti-ny fair-y's toes. Like a ti-ny fair-y's toes.

With my head held high in the morning sun,
I feel the sunshine tickle my chin.
And it makes me feel all smily,
Like a tiny fairy grin.
Like a tiny fairy grin.

## Make a Suncup

Hold your palms cupped, facing the sun so that you feel its heat and light in the center of your hands. After your hands are filled with sunlight, pour the light into your eyes. Let your eyes have a long drink of light out of your hands. End with Palming.

# Color Therapy

In the psychopharmacology department at the University of Melbourne, Trevor Norman sets depressed people under strong white light for two hours each day. Every minute they glance at the light. After two weeks their SADness (seasonal affective disorder) is relieved. He believes that the blue-green wavelength entering eyes regulates levels of the hormone melatonin. Melatonin levels increase in the evening when the sun goes down and decrease at sunrise. Daily Sunning for five minutes could have the same uplifting effect. Natural sunlight contains all color wavelengths. You will be taking in the blue-green wave while Sunning.

### 👁 Blue Lagoon

To set up a blue-green experience with your children, use theater gels or colored transparency paper from a stationery shop placed in front of an ordinary incandescent lightbulb. Or hold colored paper in front of your face while Sunning. Imagine you are in a lagoon, swimming with fishes and mermaids. You could be at the Great Barrier Reef, exploring wrecked rusty ships, finding sunken treasure.

Each color of the rainbow affects your feelings. A bright yellow room will wake you up. A blue room, especially in turquoise shades, will calm and soothe. Blue is the accepted healing color for eyes and vision. Blue skies, bluebirds, bluebells, blue frogs, can be imagined while Palming (page 106). See how color from the sun, your imagination, and your feelings all interplay.

### 👁 Prebirth Sunning

In *The Well Pregnancy Book*, Mike Samuels, M.D., recommends that expecting mamas expose their belly to direct sunlight. The effect on the baby in utero is stimulation of visual perception. At seven months all senses are receiving.

Your yet-to-be-born child hears you humming and singing, while absorbing the vibrations of light.

## Timetable for Sunning

### Birth to Two Years +

Babies and toddlers need ten minutes of sunlight daily on their skin for vitamin D production and pituitary stimulation. After that they must be completely protected by clothing and a sun hat from any degree of sunburn.

### Two to Six Years +

Two-year-olds will imitate anything, including people closing their eyes and making circles around the sun. When they are ready, voice a "thank-you" to the sun for its life-giving force. Introduce them to painting the sun different colors with total "hands-on" enthusiasm.

### Six to Twelve Years +

Circle on imaginary sunflowers with closed eyes. Invent new Sunning images together. Create a balanced rational attitude toward UV light: neither too much exposure nor too little—neither irrational fear nor disrespect for its power.

## ☙ Scared of the Dark

Many children (and adults too) are afraid of the dark. When eight-year-old Jack switched off his brain while looking at a black crayon, his whole family engaged in drawing and storytelling to resolve the issue. Jack's younger sisters had to escort him to the outdoor toilet at night. This came out as we all sat on the floor sketching with crayons on large sheets of paper. The instructions were to draw a nighttime picture on one half of the sheet and a daytime view on the other half. Jack's night side is completely covered with crayon: no images, only jet

Jack's drawing of night and day          Emma's drawing of night and day

black obscurity. His daytime drawing shows blue sky, himself, a football. By contrast his four-year-old sister's night drawing shows her house, stars, and a crescent moon. The sunny-day side is drawn completely in yellow crayon, with a boat riding on yellow waves. What is fascinating is her name: the first letters *E* and *m* are drawn in black; the following *m* and *a* are in daylight yellow. She is at peace with the duality of day and night within herself.

I suggest doing the drawing game of day and night with all children. If any fears are expressed verbally or with black crayon, do the Melting Beach Balls games. (For a full explanation of this procedure, see page 119.)

| **Positive** | **Negative** |
|---|---|
| I love the light. | I'm afraid of the light. |
| I love the darkness. | I'm afraid of the dark. |

Place the phrase "I love the light" in your left hand. Imagine a large yellow beach ball in your palm. Repeat the words "I love the light." Allow your memories about the sun coming up in the morning and illuminating the world to flow freely. Intensify all the feelings, either those that say, "The flowers are growing because of the light," or "Actually I hate to get up in the morning and go to school and do my chores and suffer." When you have explored your feelings about light to your satisfaction and blown your yellow beach ball up to world-class proportions, put the opposite in your right hand: "I'm afraid of the light." "The cancer lady who came to school told us it makes holes in your skin. I will go blind if I go outdoors. You must never go outdoors in the sun." (These statements came from a five-year-old after her school was visited by a well-intentioned Anti-Cancer Society lecturer.)

Once all social input and inner fears have been voiced and magnified (celebrated), then you ask the questions, "Is it okay to be afraid of the light?" and "Is it okay to love the light?" When the answer on both sides is yes, bring your two beach balls together at your heart. Do the same process using the sentences "I love the darkness" and "I'm afraid of the dark." When magnifying the beach ball you can ask the question, "What happens in the light?" or "What happens in the darkness?" to coax out any shy thought-gnomes that may feel it's not safe to show themselves. After doing Melting Beach Balls with light and dark, see if behavior alters in relationship to necessary, solitary trips into darkness. See if irrational fears about either sunlight or darkness, both of which relate to life and death themes, are softened or dissolved.

# 10

# Children Relax with Imagination and Color

## Are Children Relaxed?

Inside children with visual blur there is a room where they are tied up in knots. This room could be well hidden. Little myopes perform well in school. They laugh, make jokes, engage in sports. A hyperopic child with eye coordination problems catches up with her class when she puts on magnifying lenses. It looks as if we have a happy, well-adjusted child once she gets the correct glasses. But there's still that hidden room.

It is my hope that with the help of this book you and your child will be able to find that hidden room: open doors, unlock drawers, and sweep away stress. This is of greater value to me than knowing that your child is performing to social standards.

This chapter gives you more ideas for relaxation games that can be linked to home and school activities. Everyone's creativity, communication, and joy in living will go up a notch, as well as his or her visual acuity. Relaxing and imagining gives everyone courage and strength for opening closed rooms.

Relaxation comes from activating the right hemisphere of the brain. Relaxation does not mean collapsing and falling asleep. True relaxation is a state of dynamic softness and receptivity. Relaxed minds are natural springs of bright ideas and bubbling wit; unrestrained by competition and correction. Relaxed eyes light up. Life energy freely circulates through the whole visual system.

Engaging in a free flow of pleasant images produces relaxation. Everyone has these imaging abilities built in. It is not necessary to take a drug to visualize. The river of images will have a theme and a direction. The images are never wrong. If someone puts purple spots on an eagle and sets him down to drink dirty-sock tea with a whale in the middle of the oven, then that's the way it is. Brainstorming sessions in high-tech corporations have three rules. First, all ideas are correct; there are no scornful voices saying, "That's unrealistic." Second, wild and zany ideas are encouraged. Third, the more ideas the better. During an NVI teachers' conference, we brainstormed ways to do the Bird Swing with trees. The list reached 124 possibilities. It was difficult to stop and go home.

Please do not allow anyone to mess with imagery games using a left-brain compulsion to correct and be rational. A friend in Los Angeles asked his four-year-old where kangaroo mothers carry their babies. She replied, "In their mouth." Dad chided, "No, you know better than that. Kangaroos carry their babies in their pouch." Tracey had never seen a kangaroo. Her dad had never seen our local endangered frog that carries its babies in its mouth.

If your child is already caught up in the habit of worrying, if she projects negative futures, the following games will be most helpful. This child could use a story that both addresses her inner nervousness and helps her gain control of her imagination. All children need skills to accept and change the images parading through their minds. Children are open receivers. They witness adult soap operas at home and on the screen. They read books and talk to other children. By the age of six, youthful memory banks are crowded with video store categories: horror, comedy, romantic drama, action chases, science fiction, war documentaries. These films need to be coaxed out, reviewed, transmuted, and defused if your child is being controlled or affected by them.

## Home Again in the Self

A child who respects and uses her imagination becomes very independent. You as an adult may have to get used to going inside your own head in order to meet the child who is already in hers. Imagination has been schooled out of most adults. When did you stop drawing? At what age did you stop writing stories? You can regress back to that stage and start up again with painting pictures in your mind. Never mind if your paints are all dried up.

If parents are too busy to laze around with their child or to take fifteen minutes for a heart-to-heart talk, children will seek stimulation or anesthesia elsewhere. Television sets have become baby-sitters and pseudoentertainers. The amount of time children spend watching television means they are not spending time with their own life process.

Television becomes a substitute for personal imagination and sharing inner worlds. If a child has an active inner life that is shared with the world at large, watching TV will be too boring. Replace some of your child's TV watching time with your time. Let the housework or golf game go.

## Imagining with Palming

Palming is an ancient technique for healing eyes. I can see the Flintstones lying around a fire pit, Palming and telling dinosaur stories. Yogis have been Palming their eyes for several thousand years. I don't know what pictures they had going through their minds!

What is Claire imagining?

Palming sends healing energy from warm hands into eyes and mind. When Palming you have nowhere else to go except inside yourself. Shutting off all outside light stimulation rests retinal cells and gives you a break from the obligations of the outside world. Most people think that imagining does not affect the visual system. The latest in scientific research confirms that the opposite is true. When you imagine a horse running across the plains, your foot kicking a ball, or the smell of a red rose, electricity and blood circulation increase in your visual brain. Generating internal images causes bodily changes. This fact is used constantly in Natural Vision Improvement to relax muscles, establish fusion, and generally restore brilliant, clear eyesight.

### How to Palm

Cup your hands and place them over your eyes so that all outside light is shut out. I like to close my eyes under my palms. Then you do your best to turn off thinking and turn on your inner movies. You can do this alone or you can make a Palming Circle with friends.

### Palming Variations

- Someone read a book while others are Palming.
- Someone start a story and pass it to the next person.
- Someone choose a color; everything imagined has to be in that color.
- Someone choose a theme such as animals or sports. All the participants have to tell about an animal or game they are seeing in their own mind.

- Smells will bring out memory pictures in your mind faster than anything else. One person gather some smelly things together and hold them under the nose of the person who is Palming. Suggestions: fresh grass, a flower, vanilla essence or some cooking oil on tissue paper, some cinnamon or soap. Ask the question, "What does this smell remind you of?"

Carina reads a story for her Palming Circle.

- Combine sketching with Palming. As images rise up behind your closed eyes, sketch them with your Magic Nose Pencil. This will bring together movement and relaxation.

- Draw a big house inside your mind containing lots of different kinds of food for different sorts of animals. What kind of food do you have in your house? Hay? What sort of animal would like to come in the door and eat that hay? What sound does this animal make? Take turns with this game.

# Autosuggestion Training

Used by psychologists, psychiatrists, and producers of meditation cassettes, autosuggestion consists of repeated verbal phrases that deliberately release muscles and deepen breathing. The autonomic nervous system responds instantly to autosuggestion. Cold hands and feet turn warm; a mild tingling sensation is felt; contracted muscles lengthen. Child therapist and counselor Else Mueller has written books to read to children at bedtime. Her stories are framed by autosuggestions, and the characters within the story are taken through a process of relaxation—including the elves and frogs. I would add Palming to the process.

## Bedtime Story

Everyone lie down except the person who is reading slowly and soothingly. Use the following suggestions before each bedtime story. Your child's arms may come down and hands fall away from her face. That's okay. Sleep comes quickly. If you tell a story during the day when melatonin levels are close to zero, an older child will relax deeply while her mind stays alert.

> Your legs are growing very long. Your back is relaxed and long. Feel how heavy your body is. Your arms are getting long. Your arms are lighter than air. They float upward and bend at the elbows, so your hands fall gently over your closed eyes. All the light is closed out. It's like going into a warm, soft cave where everything is dark. Here comes a story.

## The Ugly Duckling Story

Mother Duck proudly looked over the five white eggs in her nest beside the pond. Every day she spread her warm brown feathers over them and closed her eyes, dreaming of the cute little yellow ducklings that would soon follow her down to the water to swim. One morning after nibbling on grass blades and swallowing a black beetle, Mother Duck returned to her nest to dream again of her new family. She did not notice the sixth egg that was nestled among the others. Ducks can only count to five.

On a dewy spring morning, Mother Duck woke up and lifted one orange foot high in the air. She had heard a cracking sound. The first duckling was pecking his way through the eggshell. Mother duck waddled off her nest.

With happy eyes she watched bits of eggshell flying in all directions. Her babies were hatching. She clucked and clicked and chuckled. She wanted her ducklings to hear her voice first so they would always come when she called. Mother Duck wriggled her white tail feathers over their heads so they would learn the shape of her rear end and always follow her when she moved. The soft morning sun dried the ducklings' wet downy feathers. Each duckling turned into a cute yellow ball of fluff with precious little orange legs and alert, beady eyes.

All except the sixth duckling. When she was sun-dried her feathers were dull gray. Her legs were long and clumsy. Her eyes rolled around in all directions. Mother Duck turned her head from side to side as she scanned this duckling. She wondered if this one really belonged in her family. Deciding that a duckling is a duckling no matter what color or what size it is, Mother Duck waddled down to the water's edge. Five cute ducklings and one ugly duckling followed her white tail feathers and her quacking voice right into the water for their first swim.

The next day other animals and the farmer's children came round to see the freshly hatched ducklings. They *oooh*ed and *aaah*ed over the five cute fluffy ducklings with their little orange feet. They frowned and threw stones and sticks at the gray, google-eyed duckling.

The Ugly Duckling let her head droop. She wandered away from the nest, shedding big hot tears from her sad eyes. "Nobody loves me," she said to the empty blue sky. "Nobody wants me," she moaned in the cool black night. "I'm terribly ugly," she screamed at the silent hard sun.

The Ugly Duckling wandered alone over hills, down roads, through cities, across fields. Everywhere people said, "Scat!" Animals said, "Shoo!" The trees and flowers said nothing.

Winter came, snowflakes fell from the sky. The Ugly Duckling shivered by a pond covered with a thick layer of ice. She let her wings droop. Her shoulders softened. She closed her eyes. She imagined warm summer sun stroking her feathers. Feel how heavy her body became. She sank into the ground. At the same time she grew bigger until she filled the whole sky. Her breathing became very slow; feel her long deep breaths.

She looked upward into softly falling snow. One snowflake grew wings— great white wings that flapped and made a wind on her face. The huge bird that owned these snow white wings landed right next to her. The Ugly Duckling was afraid to speak to such a beautiful large bird. "Hello," said the graceful, long-necked swan. "I saw you down here by yourself. Can't imagine why you'd be alone at a time like this. Just when the coldest weather is coming. Where's your nest? Where's your family? What's your name? What kind of fish swim in this pond? What's the matter? Cat got your tongue?" The Ugly Duckling could only say, "*Aughh*" Her voice was rusty from not being used. "*Aughh*," she croaked. "Me. Ugly. Duckling. Google-eyes."

The beautiful swan flapped her wings, turned around three times in the mud on her strong black legs, and laughed. "You, ugly? That's funny. What a joke. Here, tickle me again tight under my wing. *HO HA*. You are one of the more handsome of us, I would say. Go have a look in the pond."

The Ugly Duckling peeked shyly into the glassy surface of the water. She turned her head from side to side. She saw a long white neck, two straight eyes, and strong white wings. "Am I you?" She asked the swan. "Am I big and gorgeous like you?" "Yes, yes, yes," said the big friendly swan. "Come along now and meet the others. You can join our nest and cuddle up with the rest of us. It's going to be a chilly black night."

## Color All Your Life

Imagining with Palming improves eyesight. Imagining colors while Palming will make cone phones ring. Color is made in our minds. There is no color in the outside world, just light beams from the sun or artificial lights bouncing around in space. The same cone phones that register color wavelengths also tell the visual brain about sharp details. If you are able to imagine color in your mind, you will perceive color and details more easily when your eyes are open.

With your eyes closed, make a noise and ask yourself and everyone else what color the noise is. See that color in your mind. Repeat the process. Listen to music and make the music into colors.

## Emotional Healing for Imagining

Is being imaginative safe? One powerful reason that children cut off their imagination is out of fear. A good many of these fears can be traced to the method of education or picked up from parents. For example:

If I imagine too much . . .

No one will like me.
I will go crazy and be taken away to the loony bin.
I will be different from everyone else, I won't fit in.
I will not give the answers the teachers want.
My dad won't love me.

As a family, explore everyone's fears about being wildly imaginative. In the business world creative imaging and wild fantasizing are called lateral thinking. People who dare to do it are well paid. Use Melting Beach Balls on page 119 to tame your fear of unbridled imagination.

## Scary Stories

Saying no to your child when she wants to watch horror movies is your prerogative. But please do not ignore the fact that she probably already has a few in her head. The following imagery games may be useful in this case. Some children remain eternally silent about what scares them the most. Frightening images control children if they are not brought out in the open. Nightmare-causing memories can be disarmed with the following activities.

## What Happens Next?

Everyone lies down and Palms. The leader asks this question: "What is the scariest thing you can think of?"

When everyone has responded, the leader asks, "What's the worst thing that can happen?"

When replies are flowing, keep the questions going: "Yes, and what happens next? . . . and after that what happens?"

Often this spontaneous and uncensored moviemaking will reveal surprising, maybe shocking images. Be careful not to judge. Today's children are plugged into a culture that does not monitor their minds for damage. It's up to you to give them the tools, even if you think they are "too young" to be dealing with certain images. If monsters arise, play the Sculpting Monsters game. Two can play; three or more will add to the action.

## Sculpting Monsters

Continue Palming and drawing all the images that come into your mind with your Magic Nose Pencils. Start a cooperative monster creation. One person might begin with, "I see a leg. This leg is like a tree trunk, only it is orange and covered with hairs and warts. It is stomping around by itself, moaning, 'Where is my arm?'" The next person adds an arm to the monster, a horrible arm. A third person could contribute a head or heads. After the monster is sculpted, the important decision has to be reached: What do we do with the monster? Brainstorm this question.

*Do we sprinkle holy water over it so it melts away? Do we make friends with it and ask it to dinner? Shall we enter into and become the monster, to experience what it's like in there? (It could be sad and lonely.) What about chopping it to pieces and eating it with strawberry sauce?*

You may give your child some suggestions to make it okay to resolve monsters, but the final solution must be hers. Ask her if she is satisfied at the end. If she isn't, have her spend some time with this question and give you the answer later. It may come in her dreams. Children who have nightmares can benefit greatly by being given a few conscious tools to use in their dream state. When confronted by scary images, they can take control in their dream by turning to the monster and saying, "What are you doing here and what do you want?"

Sing "The World Is a Wonder" to restore a sense of appreciation about everything you see.

## Timetable for Colors and Imagining

### Birth to One Year +

When given a color choice, most young children will choose red. If you are playing vision games with a purpose, such as favoring the phoria in strabismus (page 174), make a collection of red objects: a cloth ball, a red plastic spoon, a red scarf, a red feather. Use these red objects in your directional games with the child. Red is not a requirement; your child may go for yellow or blue.

### One to Three Years +

Let the child pick out his own clothes and toys. Red again? Place red objects around the room and drape a red scarf over a picture frame. Put a red button on the tabletop. Show your child one red object, then have him close his eyes and imagine red. Ask him to go find all the red objects you've placed in the room. With an older child, have him paint the room with his red Nose Paintbrush, exclaiming when a red object pops out of the background.

### Three to Seven Years +

Have a color theme day. "Today let's paint only with blue." Finger paints are super. Have lots of paper and see what happens. Read picture books aloud. Feel free to describe the images on the page while your child Palms and paints them in her mind.

### Seven to Ten Years +

What's your favorite color? Let's make vision-game tools in this color: a magic wand with a purple ribbon; an eye patch decorated in purple; a drawing book full of purple drawings; a dress-up day in purple. Palm with purple; pick purple flowers. Use a purple Magic Pencil or a purple Magic Feather on purple noses. Palming continues. Emotional Healing for imagination may be advisable, as most adults remember they stopped drawing and visualizing at this age.

# 11

# Feelings and Eyesight

## What Do You Feel?

I don't want a lot of people to know about when I wore glasses. It was horrible. I was never really together with my friends when they played games. I always had to think about where to put my glasses.

I was frightened about them breaking and of glass going in my eye. That's funny. I am frightened about my left eye. It doesn't feel part of me. When the vision teacher did some work to use both eyes together I was frightened. Maybe I wouldn't be able to see. I don't know what seeing means. It would be very nice to see.

I wasn't very good at sports. I didn't know why. I tried very hard but sometimes I made a mistake, like in catching a ball. I just couldn't do it and it made me very unhappy. I don't remember the operation. I don't really like all those people for giving me glasses I didn't need. I was always called names too. I don't like being called names. (Eric Kiernan, Aikido teacher, speaking from his inner child)

Why do the vast majority of people who put children into glasses ignore the inner child? Perhaps their own childhood is bottled and sealed. Every child is chock-full of feelings. Vacuum-packed, childhood feelings are preserved into adulthood. Different years have different vintages. Let us devise a small game that may help every child keep his inner self ever fresh—without the canning process.

Body posture, facial expressions, free or stiff movements of limbs, and especially the look in the eyes compose a graphic nonverbal communication that comes before proper spoken language. Is this child sad, happy, irritated, bored, vivacious, angry, or scared? His eyes will tell you, if his expression is not completely locked and deadened behind glasses.

# Seven Emotions

For me the emotional health of children has more value than social correctness. The result is happy resilient adults who relate to one another in conscious empathy.

Joy and love, pain, anger, fear, sadness, apathy, and unconsciousness each have an energy vibration and a core statement that can be voiced. Everyone cycles continually through all seven emotions. When you linger too long in a vibratory feeling and thinking pattern other than joy, you develop what is called an emotional problem.

There are many shades of emotions, all variations on the major seven. Everyone's primal state is joy. Creation brings us into life on a wave of joy and love. A return to health and happiness necessitates a return journey through whatever feelings were judged and suppressed in childhood. Seeing clearly without glasses is unrestricted enjoyment of your visual system. It is normal for vision to falter occasionally. It is normal for vision to bounce back readily in the same way a small child is sad one moment and sunny the next.

## Joy

Joy verbally expresses itself as "I love that"; "Isn't that beautiful?" "That's wonderful." Joy is the state of being in love with everything all the time. Our whole system was designed to continually return to this level after flowing through the other human feelings. If joy is judged and dampened then you may feel . . .

## Pain

You are in pain if you feel less than a calm joyful appreciation about anything. Your pain can be physical, emotional, mental, or spiritual.

Pain expresses itself verbally as "It hurts." The child is blessed whose parents teach him how to accept and transmute pain, rather than anesthetize or reject it physically and mentally. "Don't cry." "It doesn't hurt." "Just get over it." Experiment with the message "Love your pain. What is it showing you?" Children are naturally adept at transmuting pain back to joy unless they learn that pain is bad and must be buried.

If pain is judged as bad (and children pick up attitudes toward pain by the time they are one year old), then the pain level is submerged and you may experience . . .

## Anger

Yes, children do get angry. Repressed anger can reemerge as hyperopia and crossed eyes. These are children who can throw champion temper tantrums. When doing vision games with these children, kindly make the room and your psyche reaction-proof. Make sure everything the child might touch is hardy. Have lots of pillows and cushions for pouncing and pounding when the urge to take action appears. "My, what a wonderful roaring lion you are!" Set limits in the midst of chaos. The first limit is the sanctity of someone else's body. "Don't hit your little sister, hit the couch." The trust that the child's life energy will bring him back to a state of tranquillity will allow you to put up with free expression of anger.

When anger is suppressed it comes out mentally as "I'm right about this and you are wrong." Some phrases heard when suppressed anger rules the personality are: "The doctors are right and everyone else, including you and your intuitive feelings, is wrong" or "There is no scientific proof and your own experience is not proof enough" or "Those blankety-blank doctors ruined my (her, his, their) eyes." Don't blame the doctors. Be angry, express it, and rise to pain and joy. Your power to act and influence reality returns.

If anger is not permitted at all, then the vibrations of the child may slow down to . . .

## Fear

Fear says or thinks, "I'm scared I will do it wrong" or "Are you sure you're doing the right thing?" or "What if we only do vision games and our child goes blind?" Myopes are constantly struggling with the fear of not being perfect in society, in school, or with friends. Myopes become masters at hiding their fear, eventually even from themselves.

If fear is not accepted and befriended, then your whole mind and body will sink into . . .

## Sadness

Sadness makes children tired if tears are not completely shed with great enthusiasm. Chronic fatigue syndrome can appear later in adolescence and adulthood. It is better to encourage full crying now, until sunbeams reemerge from behind sad, heavy clouds. Expressions of sadness find their way into left-brain time-linked utterances such as "I'll always be like this" or "He will never see clearly."

If boys and girls don't cry, then the human organism may experience . . .

## Apathy

Apathy expresses itself in thoughts or utterances such as, "You can't do that." "I'm sorry, Mrs. Smith, there is nothing that can be done about your child's eyes." "Science knows that nothing works" or "It doesn't matter." The nicest people are apathetic in their confident assurance that you just cannot change this child's vision.

If we judge and hate the apathy in others or ourselves, then we get so wiped out we fall right into . . .

## Unconsciousness

Here is the repository of all our forgotten wisdom, remedies, healing techniques. "I don't know what to do" or "My grandmother had some answer for this, but I've forgotten what she did." Here we don't feel pain any longer, or perceive much. It's a safe place to hang out but it does result in a robotic society. All anesthesias put us at this level, including the ones sold over the counter.

Unconsciousness: the walking dead, Zombieville. Most of us live here. This is the worship of technological response. Cut it out. Cover it. Drug it. Make it stop. Go to sleep. Forget about it. Deny it. It doesn't exist. It has no validity. It isn't scientific.

The only way out of the valley of unconsciousness that prevails in our "it's normal to be sick" society is to be in a state of wonder about it. Everything that exists is a miracle, no matter how awful it may appear. Then our life energy jumps right back up to joy.

A child comes into life with heaps of flexibility. He cries and then smiles, he sleeps and is ready to go again; he uses emotion as a playground. Suspend the judge.

## 👁 Eyes Talk

Eyes communicate with one another continually. This silent language can be more powerful than words. Deadness of expression in the eyes means outgoing messages have been stifled and feelings are no longer being expressed directly. When people first take off their glasses, they are not only afraid of making mistakes, they are also frightened of allowing a tear or a spark of anger to show. Take away the fear and the eyes begin to talk once more. What do they say?

Psychologists have observed the way bosses and underlings use their eyes. A manager's extended stare communicates, "I'm stronger and bigger than you." Workers avert their eyes, admitting, "I'm guilty" or "I'm intimidated." Playing a dominant role requires hiding emotions, while the subordinate player must display his nervousness and tense his shoulders and drop his head.

This scenario is enacted in offices, in classrooms, and at home. If you are aware of the game being played through silent visual communications, you have a behavior choice. You can take it seriously at the risk of all the actors getting hypnotized by their roles, or you can remark on and mime the communication gestures. Playing with eye talk will free everyone to change his or her language. If you have a goal of treating others as equals, including children, then awareness of unconscious eye and body language will bring you closer to that aim. Notice how eyes talk in your family. Your and your children's visual expression can be explored in all its subtleties and allowed to develop without fear or withdrawal. Good vision includes direct communication from eye to eye.

Everyone can develop more emotional flexibility and more time in the hall of joy by exploring candidly what comes up. To set the stage for this, you could play with recognizing and celebrating different emotional states.

## ◉ Playacting

Each person does an emotion for three to four minutes, then passes to another person, who represents another emotion.

Teach children the common words and phrases they will hear with each brand of bottled-up feeling.

| anger | "*He* did it." |
| sadness | "She *always* takes my crayon." |
| apathy | "I don't care." |
| unconsciousness | "I *forgot*. I don't remember." |

Read stories that express emotions while the children are Palming. They will be glad to contribute sound effects.

With the following emotional healing game it may be possible to help every child loosen up emotionally and stay loose. Children will seek help from you by being annoying, withdrawn, obnoxious, ill, or in a visual blur so that you will take notice, see, and help. It's not moving through the emotion that is the problem. It's getting stuck in that emotion.

##  Melting Beach Balls

In Melting Beach Balls the players celebrate negative feelings until those forbidden sensations become hilarious. This levity is the breakthrough we're looking for. You may have noticed that some children take themselves most seriously. This is where we want to uncover natural levity—a lightness of being inherent in every person. This is not teasing, ridiculing, or denying but a true celebration of what is. Often what is there is self-hate. If people disapprove of the fact that I hate myself, I will bury it even deeper with my little shovel. Once we dig up hate and take a good look at this truly unpleasant feeling and state of mind, then we can ask, "What is the opposite of hating myself?" Do not ask this latter question too early in the game or someone will think you have a preference.

### I CAN BE. . .
*Words by Janet and Donald, Music by Donald Woodward*

I can be sad, I can be mad, but___ most of the time I am filled with joy.

Da da da da, Da da da da, Yes,___ most of the time I am filled with joy.

I can be scared,
I can be brave,
but most of the time I am filled with joy.
Da, da, da, da,
Da ,da, da ,da,
Yes, most of the time I am filled with joy.

I can be blue,
I can be brown,
but most of the time I am filled with joy.
Da, da, da, da,
Da ,da, da ,da,
Yes, most of the time I am filled with joy.

**Make up your own words!!**

You may think celebrating the negative gives it power. Please realize that self-negation is already there. Because it is also unacceptable it is hidden. This develops into a psychic canker in the smallest of children. Suppressed feelings control behavior. Consider bringing out and celebrating the negative until it loses the power it has gained by being judged and closeted. Watch your child shine after his negatives have been released from the dungeon.

The following Emotional Healing game is based on embracing the opposites in life. Melting together hate and love, fear and courage, ugliness and beauty, heals the split, the separation between our left and right halves, between mind and body. If you are even slightly successful with this game, you will notice a lessening of tension in your child's body and eyes.

A child in the original state of grace doesn't choose sides in any fight. Through these games children can learn to actually manipulate fear or anger and consciously bring in states of pleasure and joy. When your children are taught this useful trick at a young age, you will find your teenagers priding themselves on how they can sit on a rock alone, resolving their own moods and problems.

## The Preliminary Game:

## Learning to Melt Opposites Together

*I'm a little angel. I'm so good. Everybody loves me.*
*I'm a little devil. I'm naughty: I'm bad. Nobody loves me.*

Put "I'm a little angel" in your right hand in a big ball of energy. Put "I'm a little devil" in your left hand in a big ball of energy. Switch back and forth, stating the message of each ball and making that ball bigger and stronger—until we sing, or whisper, or scream our message to the sky. When satisfied do. . .

## The Last Move of the Game

Squish and smoosh together slowly, passionately, your right-hand ball and your left-hand ball like Scarlett is doing in the photo opposite. Her physical beach balls won't blend together, but your imaginary ones will. They will come together like matter and antimatter; perhaps with a BANG!, a *poof*, or a *Shhhhh*. Then interlace the fingers of your two hands and bring them to the middle of your chest. Release your hands, your arms. Feel your lightness of being.

Practice filling up and expanding Beach Balls with other opposites, such as:

| | |
|---|---|
| sad | happy |
| scared | brave |
| stupid | smart |

Become skilled at melting concepts together by practicing with colors. Choose a colored crayon that feels like sad. With this color make a big circle on a piece of paper. Color in the circle so you have a beach ball of solid blue, for example. Hold the crayon in your hand and truly feel that color. Close your eyes. Is it a heavy color or a lightweight color? Now open your eyes and pick a crayon that feels like the opposite of sad. What does this color feel like? Is it heavy or lightweight? On a second sheet of paper make a solid beach ball with this crayon.

Hold your drawings in your hands, the sad color in one hand and the happy color in the other hand. Close your eyes. Imagine both balls growing huge—right off the paper.

Now bring your hands together, crumpling the paper. Imagine the colors are mixing together. What color would this be?

Open your eyes and draw a beach ball circle made of both colors on another paper. Put it on the wall and explain to your friends.

Scarlett is magnifying her Beach Balls.

Scarlett smooshes her Beach Balls together.

Scarlett releases it all!

##  Take a Deep Breath

I have included breathing and yawning in this chapter about feeling and emotion because suppressed feelings are held in place by restricted breathing. A child who freely breathes is a child whose emotions will flow quickly to a state of joy and openness. Yawning frees the breath. Yawning releases tight jaws, tummies, and eyes. Yawning brightens and clears eyesight. Yawning increases oxygen supply to eyes and brain. Free breathers are clear seers.

## Yawning with the Lions

Playact together:

A lion sits under a tree and yawns loud and lazily. He is imagining what he would like to eat. Off in the distance the lion sees something that might be delicious, but he does not recognize exactly what it is. He wants to stroll over there and find out if it would suit his tummy for dinner. The lion stretches out his long front legs, then his long back legs. He yawns again. Softly, carefully he crawls toward the other creature—on all fours of course. Silently, feeling the ground beneath his paws, he sneaks up on his dinner. Pouncing on his dinner, the lion eats it all up with groans of pleasure and mighty slurps. Yawn.

## 👁 Huff-Puff

A short, easy breathing release for children who are already tied up in knots and for all children to keep them emotionally free.

> Duration: thirty seconds.
> When: during cuddle times or at bedtime.
> Position: with the child lying flat on his back on a bed or the floor or on your lap.
> How: Place your hand lightly on your child's tummy. There is a golden balloon inside this tummy. When your child inhales, the balloon gets bigger, the tummy fatter. When he exhales, all the air in the balloon goes out. We now have a flat tummy. Do this three times. With small children that's enough. Adults have to breathe for an hour to get the same effect.
> Response: Ask him how he feels.

Tummy breathing slows down the heartbeat and stimulates a right-brain, muscle-lengthening relaxation response. Chest breathing stimulates a left-brain, hold-tight state in the body. For good, balanced breathing and brain function we need both tummy and chest movement.

## 👁 Joyful Seeing and Singing

Say to the child:

As you are growing and exploring with your eyes, ears, mouth, and fingers, the people who are caring for you play silly, silly games with you. They hang bright, shiny things above you that move in the wind. They put pictures up for you to play with, first only with your eyes, then with your fingertips. They cuddle you and sing to you. Later, you will sing these songs to yourself and with your friends. You are a vision person.

# THE GOODNESS SONG

*Words and melody by Janet Goodrich, Music by Donald Woodward*

# TELL ME WHAT YOU SEE

*Lyrics by Janet Goodrich, Music based on a prelude by Chopin*

# IF YOU'RE HAPPY AND YOU KNOW IT

*Traditional*

If you're hap-py and you know it clap your hands; If you're

hap-py and you know it clap your hands; If you're

hap-py and you know it, then you real-ly ought to show it, If you're

hap-py and you know it clap your hands.

If you're happy and you know it do cross crawl...
If you're happy and you know it swing your head...
If you're happy and you know it blink a lot...
If you're happy and you know it sun your eyes...
If you're happy and you know it yawn out loud...
If you're happy and you know it palm your eyes...
If you're happy and you know it smile a lot...

## Timetable for Emotional Expression

### Birth to One Year

Infants have feelings. Our society and upbringing call for us not to know what to do for ourselves and not to express our feelings. Learn to receive the baby's cries of anger, fear, and distress the best you can with supportive tranquillity even though you may be tired and grumpy yourself. Singing, toning, crooning, making noises with the child, help immensely. They carry your own tension away. If your jaw is tightening up and you're looking for an escape route, make noises with the kids. Hold the points described in chapter 6 on yourself and your baby. Discover how soothing and freeing it can be. Apply love, and forgiveness of self and others. Include the doctors.

### Three Years +

Act out emotions:  Do Yawning and Huff-Puff.
                   Sing vision people songs.

### Six Years +

Use Melting Beach Balls; make the eyes and faces of the seven emotions to look at while jumping on the trampoline.

# 12

# Winning Eye Tests without Glasses

The secret to winning eye tests without glasses has two parts. The first part is white, namely the Great White Glow on page 131. The Glow appears when everyone uses his or her eyes the way nature intended: easily, without straining or trying.

Eyes see by receiving light from whatever you're looking at. A red ball sends only the red wavelength to the eyes, absorbing all the other colors. White paper sends every color to your eyes. Black print absorbs all the light, sending nothing to your eyes; therefore black letters are not actually seen. We recognize the shape of a letter by the white space around it. Teaching children early to mentally tune in to the white spaces, rather than straining to see the "unseeable" black print, will prevent many problems with reading books and eye charts.

The second part of the secret is to finally recognize that eye tests are stress generators for children. Everyone should realize that eye tests are loaded with performance anxiety. This anxiety is akin to stage fright and in itself creates blur.

## The Unspoken Obligation in Eye Tests

The pressure to see is not limited to letters on flat cards. There is an obligation charge on many things that appear in our visual field. Dr. Bates observed that when people looked at a plain white background, their refractive error would lessen or disappear. When a child was being tested on an eye chart and other children were looking on, waiting to see what results Johnny came up with, Johnny went myopic. "No child wants to be stupid," said the NVI teacher and optician Helga Gryzb. She remembers her thought pattern from her first vision test at age six. In many children's minds, failing an eye test is equated with being stupid, a complete downer. Both myopic and hyperopic children register high on the obligation scale. High obligation creates stress, usually with great anticipation of failure thrown in.

| High obligation | Low obligation |
|---|---|
| • black-and-white test charts | • plain white paper |
| • Mom's face when she's angry | • clouds, bunny rabbits |
| • jeering children's faces | • friendly glowing faces |
| • words in books | • sand on the beach |

It is possible for all children to stay relaxed when reading letters in books and on eye charts. Getting both sides of the brain switched on helps; releasing test anxiety with Melting Beach Balls does wonders. In this chapter you will learn a new method of relating visually to black-and-white print. Make this method, called Painting White, a lifelong habit. See if any over-forties in your family will take off their reading glasses and join in.

## Make Your Own Eye Charts

Daniel loves his viruses and used them to make his own eye chart.

My strategy for wringing the threat out of eye charts is to have NVI students make their own. In Vision Playcamps I ask the children what their favorite themes are. Ten-year-old Anthony said soccer. Six-year-olds Jack and Margo like cuddly animals. Daniel had just seen a TV program on viruses (see his chart on page 130). Little Jack, at four, was enthralled with cars.

When the children were supplied with full-sized white poster paper and chunky black crayons, a collection of eye charts appeared. Little Jack brought his collection of *MotorCar* magazines. He cut out cars and pasted them on the poster paper. The larger cars were at the top, diminishing in size to the bottom row. Even though some of the cars were colored, Jack could still Paint White around them, calling off their names from greater and greater distances.

After making a few theme eye charts, we move to letters and numerals.

Have your child make her favorite letters on white paper with large black crayons or broad, felt-tip pens. Make letters in different sizes.

Cut the letters out and paste them on a piece of white poster paper. Hang your child's personal eye charts on the wall in the kitchen or in her room.

Mereki making her distance chart

G H Z
Q X O

You will end up with three different charts. The first one will have only shapes on it in the child's current and favorite theme. The next chart could have a mix of shapes and letters or words. Your child will be faced with the third kind, the chart with only letters on it, on school eye-testing day or at the optometrist's office. This chart comes last. Do not worry about her memorizing her charts; she will. Holding the familiar shapes in her mind and seeing them from farther away will build her confidence. When you begin Painting White games, sit at a distance from the chart where the top three lines are easy to recognize.

So far I have talked about eye charts for distance blur. Children with high degrees of myopia, hyperopia, or astigmatism may have blur at all distances. Hyperopes and astigmatics will need a small chart to hold in the hand with progressively smaller images. A myopic child with more than four diopters of correction will also need a near-point eye chart. In some cases you will be able to use a photocopier that reduces images to make the small chart. Or you can use a fine felt-tip pen and draw the progressively smaller hand cards. (The goat-and-giraffe chart is from the Corbett school.)

Daniel's virus chart

Shapes and letters eye chart

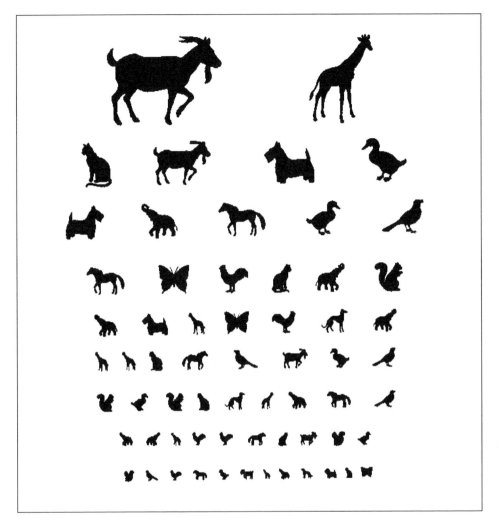

Goat and giraffe chart

##  The Great White Glow

Since our eyes don't register black ink, we want to tune in to the white spaces around the letters as a habit. Every time you glance at a black-and-white eye chart, instantly go for the white spaces. This creates high contrast between the edges of the black shapes and the white paper. Your eyes will happily dance along this sharp edge. A brilliant white glow will suddenly appear around the shape you are interested in. This is the appearance of the Great White Glow. Do the following activities to get your mind acquainted with the Great White Glow. Once the Great White Glow has shown up, repeat the games to reinforce the friendship.

### 👁 A White Thing

Begin by asking children what's white. Make a list of the answers. Do this while everyone is Palming. Then put the white things together with action words.

For example, I asked a five-year-old "What's white?" Together we wrote down the following list: snow, bird, daisy, dress, cloud, milk, doily, teeth, hair, shoes, candle, paper, waves, ice, polar bears, igloo, cream, ice cream, yogurt, ribbons, whiskers, wool goats, dove, goose, duck, pen, baby seal, in between

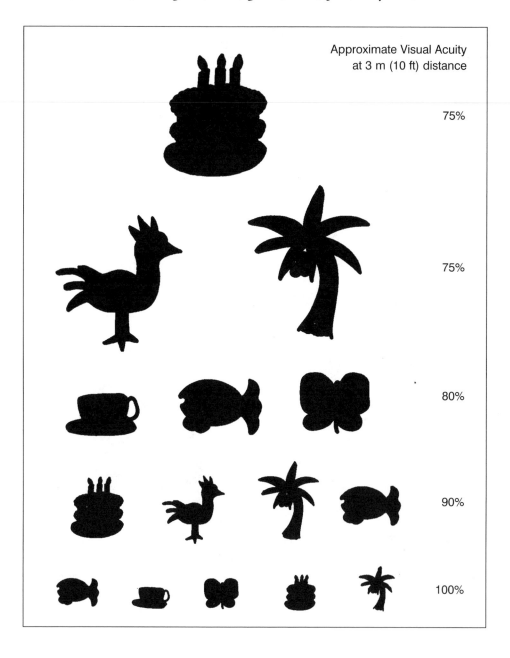

the zebra stripes, egg, horse, socks. We then glued some of the words together, obtaining zebrastripes, clouddress, milkdoily, candleteeth, creamgoose. Somehow stinkysocks got in there as well! Then we put together a little story:

> The zebra had candleteeth and stinkysocks chasing a snowhorse around an ice-creamigloo. The babyseal cried icetears and the paperwaves got real big. The ice-creamigloo melted and floated away. The duckgoose fell in the yogurt ocean and the daisybird sat on the zebra, who washed his stinkysocks in the ice cream.

At the end of conjuring up all these white pictures we definitely had white on our mind. Then we took the next step and imagined a Magic Nose Paintbrush.

## 👁 The Magic Nose Paintbrush Paints White

Pretend you have a paintbrush on the end of your nose. You can dip it in toothpaste or shaving cream and paint everything you see white. Paint the trees white, the people white, your toes white. Now let's paint white circles around the black animals and objects on the chart. Notice how the paper gets a white glow at the edges of the black. Let's close our eyes and imagine some fresh white paint on our brush. Got it? Now open your eyes and paint around the birthday cake at the top. A white glow, or aura, will appear around the birthday cake. Find more birthday cakes that glow. When surrounded by your white paint, the black shapes will become blacker. When the white is whiter and the black is blacker, you see the objects more clearly. The Great White Glow is here!

## 👁 Fishing and Finding

Rather than having your child look at blurry letters and then try to tell you what they are, let her find the letter shapes in her brain first with eyes closed, then paint white all over the chart with eyes open until that letter or shape jumps out at her. Whimsy helps banish the obligation factor. Encourage free association with the letters on the chart. For example, the chart that Felicity is using has an *O* and an *E* on it. Close your eyes. Imagine an O. Got it? Open your eyes and paint white around the O.

Aerro with his Magic Paintbrush

Felicity does Cross-Crawl, Paints White, and goes whimsical with her eye chart

Solomon can Paint White and go Fishing with his animals and their names.

O: Oh what a beautiful round doughnut. Become the O, scan, swing it around, Odel odel ehihu.

CheeriOs, OKs, UFOs, O my, O gosh, O goodness, O my darling, O dear, what can the matter be?

Oh what a beautiful mOrning. An O in the snOw. Say hellO to the O in the back of yOur nOse. Oink.

Close your eyes. Imagine an E. Got it? Open your eyes and paint white around the E.

E: East of E Street, an Emporium that sElls EvErything.

A prEEning white Emu is rEEling around an ElEgant Egg.

Eyes sEE clEarly. ThrEE vEry clEan fEEt fEEl cosy in grEEn socks.

Don't worry, painting white over black objects and letters does not erase them. In fact a lot of white paint falls through the black ink; the rest piles up along the edges like snowbanks.

Record of eye movements while reading a Shakespeare sonnet (in Russian)

# What Is Reading?

Reading can be a great joy, as messages picked up by the eyes are translated in the brain into colorful sagas of adventure and intrigue. Reading also has its shady side.

Myopes can become compulsive readers, missing out on life altogether. I taught myself to read at age four and out of my fear of the world of people I became one of those readers under the covers. At age twenty-four I realized what I was doing and did not read anything for a year. I had to pull myself away from the print on cereal boxes and newspaper headlines. Old habits. Now my life is too full to be satisfied with surrogate adventures.

Hyperopes can end up avoiding reading like the plague. Unpleasant experiences with reading in school, having to read in front of remorseless children, results in permanent allergic reaction to the printed word! Neither of these has to happen with our children if we can take a whole-brain, full-being approach to reading.

When reading, your eyes dance along the words in the pattern seen on page 134.

Eye muscles must be fully relaxed to allow this rapid movement and clear foveal vision. The right brain sends in a message of mobility and release to the eye muscles. The left brain is consciously aware of the meanings of the words. The memory aspect of reading is both short- and long-term. Can you tell me what you just read? Could you tell me next week, without peeking at this page? If you could, then you have put this message into your right brain by translating the words into images.

## Paint White

Relaxed reading with understanding and memory can be accomplished with the use of the Magic Paintbrush. Put your Paintbrush on the end of your nose and Paint White from left to right, through line one on page 136. Paint right over the black words, which will reassert themselves. Blink easily, breathe, and go on with your Paintbrush through the second line. Let the Great White Glow appear. Continue to the bottom. After you have practiced with this story, get one of your favorite books and practice painting with your Magic Nose Paintbrush through every line.

# 1 Geminy Boots

# 2 ran home from school

# 3 with a green frog in his hand

## 4 His father said to him

## 5 put that frog back in the pond

### 6 Geminy Boots ran in the rain

#### 7 His frog never left him

8 It even slept in his bed

9 and ate oats for breakfast

The Geminy Boots story can be used to assess near point vision. If you read line 9 holding the page about thirty-six centimeters (fourteen inches) away from your eyes, you have 6/6 (20/20), 100 percent close vision. Reading line 8 means you have 6/12 (20/40), 80 percent close vision, adequate for Transition Glasses. Learn this song to saturate your mind with whiteness. Music will help you keep white in mind while reading all books, papers, and eye charts.

# I LIKE PAINTING WHITE

*Words and Music by Donald Woodward*

# Emotions and Reading

Here are some thoughts and fears around reading alone or aloud in front of others:

> I will get laughed at.
> I will sound funny.
> I will not be able to keep up with the other kids.
> I am stupid.
> My eyes hurt.
> I can't breathe.
> I won't understand the words.

Ask your child. Listen for her thoughts, her fears. Play Melting Beach Balls (page 119). Have her state her fear about reading and make it an energy ball in one hand. Repeat it aloud, in all kinds of ways: loud, soft, with eyes closed and open, in a high voice, in a low voice. Make the ball bigger, give it a color. Expand it to the ceiling, to the clouds. Tell everyone in the whole world about it.

Satisfied? Ask her, "What is the opposite of being laughed at?" Listen for the answer and help her put it in the other hand. Build it up, announce it to the birds and all the animals everywhere. Tell it to the fishes in the sea. Make this ball into a color and expand it until the stars can feel it.

Now, with passion, have her squish the two balls together before releasing them. Continue reading with the Magic Nose Paintbrush and the Great White Glow.

Part 3

# Specific Programs for Specific Problems

# 13

# Myopia

## What Is Myopia?

When a child is myopic he will have blur in the distance and clear vision up close. If the myopia is severe, he may have to hold objects within centimeters (inches) of his nose to see them clearly. In Australia this child is called shortsighted; in America he is called nearsighted.

The only representation of myopia found in school textbooks and popular magazines is an elongated eyeball. The abnormal length of a myopic eyeball drops the light beams from what you are looking at onto a point in front of the macula lutea. This means no clear central vision, no sharp edges on objects far away.

One millimeter of elongation of the optical axis of the eye produces three diopters of myopia.

Pseudo- or false myopia also exists. One awakens seeing the sign at the corner clearly. After a day at work, the sign is blurry. Direct explanations for pseudomyopia are scarce, but fatigue is a factor.

My high school biology book did not address the question of how eyeballs get too long. It simply showed a minus, concave lens placed in front of this strange organ. I wondered, "If eyeballs can get longer, why can't they get shorter?"

They can—if visual habits are changed.

When the eyeball is too long, the image falls in front of the retina.

A concave lens corrects for an eyeball that is too long.

## When Does Myopia Start?

For many years myopic careers were started at age seven. More girls than boys became myopic at adolescence. By the time these children were eighteen, their myopia leveled off and stayed the same the rest of their lives.

This pattern has changed. Nowadays people at age twenty-four produce myopia for the first time—often at university or with a new job in a bank.

Some folks love the idea of teaching their children to read in the cradle. It's an enticing notion because precocious children are greatly admired, but some of these children become myopic at age four. A few mothers who have diligently homeschooled their bespectacled offspring glower at me resentfully when I mention a possible link between infants' reading and refractive error. I love the idea of homeschooling. But if left-brain training is taking place that early, it needs balancing with right-brain vision games—and plenty of them. I used to think it would be great to have a seven-year-old graduate from high school; my values have shifted.

What can we do for the child of seven or ten who is already dependent on glasses? Lots. With myopia it's not enough to throw glasses away. Vision games need to be played and inner feelings addressed.

If your myopic child is using a low prescription (under two diopters), it may be possible to park his glasses in a drawer. If he is dependent on artificial correction to see the board at school, Transition Glasses, or T-Glasses, are called for.

## Transition Glasses for Young Myopes

Your goal is to allow your child's vision to improve through the activities in this book while periodically stepping down the power of his glasses. Myopes, when they are not using lenses, experience flashes of clear sight. At first flashes last half a second, then for longer periods. A twelve-year-old NVI student whispered to me after her vision class, "My mum wanted me to tell you that I had a six-hour flash." I thanked her for telling me.

Most myopes can read easily without glasses unless they have significant astigmatism. Why then do myopes read with their specs? It is both from habit and because they have been told to.

For the purposes of this program we want children to be without glasses as much as possible so that the vision games can take effect. When they do need to set spectacles upon their noses, let it be with a minimum prescription. General guidelines for T-Glasses that you can take to your practitioner are on pages 23–25. Pin-holes can also be used as T-Glasses for myopic vision.

If your child's prescription is below two diopters (my last pair of

Transition Glasses for myopia were three and a half diopters), send a note to school asking all teachers to allow this child to sit in the front row. Give a copy of this book to his teacher. Vision games that help myopia also boost learning. Relaxed humans learn quickly.

With the requested strength of correction in the T-Glasses, your myopic child should be able to identify the letters and shapes below from a distance of six meters (twenty feet).

## Think Twice about Surgery

Relatives who read the newspaper said to myopic Michael, "Why go to that course? Just get yourself a sixteen-second operation and you'll see well enough." Radial keratotomy (Radial-K, or RK) will grow in popularity in the next decades. You could wait until your young myope turns eighteen and send him to an ophthalmic surgeon.

An advertisement in a San Francisco subway asked: "Would you like to wake up in the morning with 20/20 vision?" Yes, of course, but where is the small print? I collect it on RK. In 1985 writers of the *Harvard Health Letter* shifted their position on RK from guarded optimism to guarded pessimism. "Between one and four years after the operation, only six percent of the treated eyes retained the correction achieved by the operation." In 1988 *Consumer Reports* magazine told us the U. S. Air Force will not accept anyone who had undergone the operation. "Many of the patients are bothered by glare at night and experience some fluctuations in their visual acuity."

Techniques improve for shortening the myopic eyeball. Currently you can have epithelia (skin cells) blazed off the front of your eyeball by laser. Problems still remain. It takes four to five years for the cornea to heal fully; during this time the eyes are subject to infections. Sixteen percent of the eyes operated upon end up hyperopic; they overreact. Dr. Walter Stark, director of corneal services at Johns Hopkins School of Medicine stated, "Only a handful of ophthalmologists out of 13,000 have had the operation on themselves. If it were a simple cure-all as advertised, more would have had it. . . . You're talking about operating on a structurally normal eye with an unpredictable outcome."

Radial keratotomy does not touch the *cause* of myopia.

# What Myopia Feels Like Inside

Myopes walk on eggshells. Their sensitivity and fear of failure are frosted with capability illusions. Myopes become tough guys, debonair devils, or class clowns. If you do scratch the frosting and a state of fear appears, do not attempt to console a myope by reminding him of how many trophies he has hanging on the wall. His distress is internal. External ribbons, badges, and certificates of achievement are impressive, but they do not heal.

Young myopes feel compelled to be perfect in the eyes of others. But they remain imperfect in their own eyes. The way to help these children transmute their internal pressure is to do Emotional Healing on the issue.

## Emotional Healing for Myopia

Sit down together in a quiet place where you will not be disturbed. Use the following thought patterns to start inflating Melting Beach Balls (page 119). After a bit of practice your child will begin to present his own findings, the launching pads for his emotional rockets.

| | |
|---|---|
| Nobody loves me. | Everybody loves me. I love myself. |
| Everything I do must be perfect. | I am loved even when I screw up. |
| I hate making mistakes. | I love making mistakes. |

You and your child put the sentence "Nobody loves me" in your right hands. As you repeat the phrase, let memories and associations arise. Talk about it. Keep building up the size, color, and weight of the energy Beach Ball in your right hand. Thoroughly explore the reality of this phrase, of this belief (even if adults try to deny it), until you are totally satisfied that you have told the wind and the world about it, that it is okay that nobody loves you, because you can still love yourself (this is the secret ingredient).

Go to the opposite thought: "Everybody loves me." Somehow this is also true. Even the bully at school loves you, so does the girl who always whispers behind your back. Put the words, the thought, the feeling "everybody loves me" in your left-hand Beach Ball. Build it up to the stars, trumpet it through the galaxy. When you are satisfied with both your Beach Balls, when they are somehow equal to one another, thunder-clap them together. Lightning flashes; the whole issue flutters away.

## The Myopia/Hyperopia Connection

Myopia and hyperopia are like brother and sister: masculine and feminine aspects of sight. As your child is growing, it is completely natural for his vision to fluctuate between myopia and hyperopia.

Gesell's researchers peered into infants' eyes with a retinoscope from one meter (about three feet) away. I am paraphrasing Gesell's report and conclusions:

> A rattle was waved at fifteen feet. As the four-month-old child's eyes sought the noisy visual target, his eyes brightened and showed a myopic response. When his attention settled and held to the rattle, his eyes went hyperopic. As his attention relaxed, there was an oscillation between myopic and hyperopic response.
>
> The eye, like the hand, is an organ of manipulation, and both are governed by the cortical brain. In the last analysis it is the brain that appropriates the outer world, whether manually, orally, or ocularly. It does so by a projectile process, but this is a two-way reciprocating process—a directional process that emanates from within the self, goes out, and then returns within. The taking-in and giving-out process has a direct correlation to hyperopic and myopic states.
>
> When the child is older, his near visual tasks become more symbolic, but the retinal manifestations and the cortical (brain) demands are not profoundly different. The eye still functions as a prehensory and manipulatory organ. The preschool child's identification of a picture or a letter in a book is comparable to the infant's [grasping] and manipulation of a toy. The preschool child of three years looks for a familiar picture, and since he knows

what he is looking for, the retinoscope shows a sustained [myopic state]. The organism is "taking in" something—a visual kind of interjection. Presently the child extends arm and index finger and points to the picture; thereby he moves into the reciprocal outgoing phase of a circular cycle of response. Having "taken in," he is now projecting externally . . . the retinoscope shows a shift toward hyperopia.

Myopes and hyperopes reflect right- and left-brain imbalances, and they create distinct personality traits.

Myopes know a lot. They inhibit their impulses. They project inward rather than outward. Help young myopes unfreeze, expand, release themselves to love and imperfection.

Because myopia and hyperopia are two sides of the same coin, I suggest you read the following chapter on hyperopia. I emphasize close-to-far games in this chapter to help myopes take relaxation into the distance, but do feel free to use games from the following chapter for your myopic child.

## Reversing Myopia with NVI

*A note to parents:* Even though all vision games are useful for myopia, emphasize the following games. ("You" refers to the child.)

### Cross-Crawl Dancing (page 63)

Switch on your right brain for your eyes. Yes, it may already be switched on for your mind and body. We need it "on" for your visual system (page 61).

### The Magic Nose Pencil (page 75)

A Magic Pencil is essential for changing the myopic stare back into fast and loose saccadic movement (page 69). "Penciling" becomes your new habit and you do it while watching TV, using your computer—all the time, including when you're using T-Glasses.

### Palming (page 106)

Palm whenever your eyes feel tired: go see the movies in your head. Palm when you wake up in the morning, just before sleeping, at your desk. Make what you have just read into images for long-term memory. Then facts will stick in your brain like peanut butter to the roof of your mouth.

### Sunning (page 98)

Sun once a day or whenever you can sneak it in. Sunglasses are not that cool; high light tolerance is (page 98).

### Great White Glow (page 131)

To see eye charts clearly as well as the board at school and the score at the football game, do Painting White with the Great White Glow at least twice a week (pages 135 and 131).

When reading books, make sure you sweep through the lines on the page with your White Paintbrush. Blink and yawn while reading. Do the same when you are planted in front of a computer (page 212).

### The Fishing Rod Story

Palm while listening to the following story. Paint the images that arise in your mind with your Magic Nose Paintbrush. This tale will help extend your clear vision into the far distance:

> Lake Eyre is a huge, dry salt lake in South Australia. Every twenty years or so it fills with water after heavy rains. Thousands of pelicans and other birds go there to feed. After a few days the lake is dry again.
>
> Derjundi is an Aboriginal boy who lives near Lake Eyre. He wrote letters to his pen pal Dennis, who lives in Minnesota in North America. Minnesota is called the land of ten thousand lakes. Dennis had caught the biggest rainbow trout of the year. He sent a photo of himself sitting in his rowboat, surrounded by fishing tackle and grinning from ear to eat. For Derjundi's tenth birthday, Dennis's family bought a shiny aluminum fishing pole with reel, wrapped it carefully, and sent it by mail to Australia. When the long cardboard box arrived at Derjundi's home in the desert four months

later, his brothers and sisters jumped up and down with excitement.

The first thing Derjundi saw inside the box was green wrapping paper covered with pictures of leaping trout. "That's not the present," he announced, and ripped the paper off to reveal a glistening fishing pole. It had racing stripes painted on the rod and a cork handle. A fat reel of nylon fishing line and three large metal hooks fell out of the box. "Whatever can you do with that?" wondered Derjundi's sisters and brothers.

"They must have thought you live by a lake with water in it," yelled his little brother.

Derjundi shook his head. His father took the green paper and studied the pictures of rainbow trout.

After the flat horizon of Lake Eyre sliced the evening sun and ate it like toast, Derjundi walked out of his house with his fishing rod in hand. Kneeling in the crunchy sand, Derjundi carefully put the three lengths of the rod together. He wound the nylon line into the reel, just as it showed in the instruction book. He fastened a hook to the end of the line and sat down at the edge of Lake Eyre, waiting. His sisters and brothers ran home past him, laughing and pointing.

"He's going to catch a lot of dust devils and willy-willies."

Derjundi sat quietly for a long time, swinging his head back and forth across the millions of stars in the clear, black sky. He stood up, flung his arm back, and cast his fishing line into the sky. He heard the nylon line sizzle as it shot straight out from his fishing pole into the night sky. The sound stopped. Derjundi tugged on his rod. The line was stuck; Derjundi tugged harder and harder. He realized he had to turn the handle on the reel. He turned it, and turned it more. The line moved and slid back onto the reel. Far off in the distance Derjundi could see something wriggling on the end of his line. It was silver and shiny like a flip top from a metal soft-drink can. "I must keep reeling it in," he thought. The silver, wriggly thing finally lay at Derjundi's feet, dangling from the end of his fishing line. He edged it with his Magic Nose Pencil and blinked at it and closed his eyes to remember if he had ever seen anything like it before. He had never seen anything exactly like this. He opened his eyes and whispered, "You're a star."

With the star safe inside his fishing bag, Derjundi jogged back home. He let his brothers and sisters and cousins have a peek at the star inside his bag. "Tomorrow night I'll catch a supernova," he announced to everyone.

### Timetable for Myopia Games

**Birth to One Year +**

Rocking and swinging, massage, and Holding Points

**One to Three Years +**

Cross-Crawl dancing

**Three to Five Years +**

Palming and Near-Far Swings

**Five to Ten Years +**

Magic Nose Pencil, Palming, Painting White and the Great White Glow, Nuclear Vision games, and Painting Pictures game

# 14

# Hyperopia

## What Is Hyperopia?

An eyeball that is too short is hyperopic. Blur results when viewing close objects. The short axial length of the eyeball causes the light beams from what you are looking at to fall behind the retina. A person could be so hyperopic that his or her blur range extends from up close to into the landscape. The physical aspect of hyperopia is compensated for by placing magnifying (plus) lenses in front of the eye.

The shortened eyeball lets the image fall behind the retina.

At birth most infants' eyes are hyperopic. By adolescence these short eyeballs should stabilize at the normal axial length, creating a state called emmetropia, which means normal vision. For this reason, eye doctors tell parents, "She may outgrow it. But have her wear these glasses in the meantime when she is reading."

This approach encourages parents to put hyperopic children in glasses and wait to see what happens. Duke-Elder states that 50 percent of hyperopic children do in fact grow out of the condition; the other half end up as hyperopic adults in magnifying lenses.

## Many Children Outgrow Hyperopia

Optical professionals who find hyperopia with retinoscopy will recommend plus lenses for the child even when she can see clearly at all distances. Parents wonder why she should use glasses when she has no trouble seeing. The reasoning goes like this: Accommodation is the ability of the lens of the eye to change its curvature. When you look at a tree on the far hill, your lens flattens. Glancing at the time on your watch causes ocular muscles to tighten and the lens to bulge, gathering in the light from your watch face to place it on

A convex lens compensates for an eyeball that is too short.

your macula lutea. If a child has strong lens accommodation (and most children do), she will be able to use this ability to focus on everything clearly, including her book. For this reason, when asked, "Why should she wear spectacles?" the optical specialist replies, "Because she is using her accommodation ability to compensate for her too-short eyeballs. And if she does not use the magnifying lens I'm prescribing for her, her eyes are going to get very sore and tired from overaccommodating."

I would rather give this child relaxation tools: Palming for tired eyes and Painting White for effortless reading. My experience with hyperopic adults and children has shown that hyperopia is easy to dissolve with Natural Vision Improvement when the student is willing.

## What Hyperopia Feels Like Inside

Hyperopic children are often wild cards, tantrum throwers, cross-eyed little demons, awkward misfits. In a recent Playcamp, five myopic instructors were matched to five hyperopic children. Two 1.8-meter (6-foot) male teachers had to forsake their carefully laid activity plans. The wee hyperopes were moving too fast. Not all hyperopic children bring pandemonium in their wake. Some are petite feminine dictators who run the show disguised as fairy princesses.

Hyperopic children are teachers come to jolt adults out of their conventions, out of their pedestrian trance. They are usually misunderstood. Their fantasies and insights have no precedent; teachers can't find their responses in textbooks. They must be wrong. Some hyperopes learn quickly and early to keep their right-brain antics well under control. Others blow you away with their explosions, demands, and insights. I think these children contain yet-to-be discovered solutions to world problems.

Hyperopes react to school desks like tigers to cages. *Why can't she sit still?* Even if the tiger is externally calm, an inner revolt is simmering. Anger is swallowed to cope with society. When grown-up, this girl may become an overdirective and strict music teacher.

Many hyperopes are on watch, playing eternal guard duty. NVI teacher Gloria Veit writes about her hyperopic childhood:

It's possible that myopes are church mice with squeaky voices. That does not mean that I, as a hyperope, feel like a cat stalking those mice to eat them up. I feel more like the dog that looks after everything and everybody, making sure that no strangers get too close. I actually guard the church mice. Sometimes while playing with a delicate mouse my paws come down too heavily on her tail.

If I look around and see any injustice being done, I will howl. If anyone tries to cage me, I will bite hard. I'm the fighter, the controller, and the captain. I want to guard the world so it doesn't dissolve in chaos. Otherwise all the details will fly at me, penetrate my protective distance, pushy and invasive. Pushiness is something hyperopes can't stand. If someone comes too close to me, I can't breathe.

I assume that every hyperope carries around a secret wound, a basic fear of love. As a tiny child I felt that if I gave myself completely to love, someone would destroy it, the most precious thing in my life. So I decided to bury this precious jewel deep inside myself, so deep I forgot where it was. I'd be afraid to dig it out anyway. I convinced myself that people who love completely abandon themselves to pain. Anger is stuck in me. I'm stuck in anger. I was bitterly, angrily disappointed as a child when my love was rejected. Suppressing this anger made me strong, gave me a defense against the encroachment of others, and kept me from having to resurrect my love. (Translated from German by Janet Goodrich)

## Emotional Healing for Hyperopia

The hyperopic child is missing self-love and refuses to get close to others or herself. This tendency lasts into adulthood. Hyperopic adults who search within find a small child who's angry at the world. She tells everyone to bug off and leave her alone. But this is not really what she wants. Her life energy pushes her to seek tumultuous and awkward contact. Use Melting Beach Balls (page 119).

These are the general thought patterns of our small hyperopic friends:

| | |
|---|---|
| Go away. | Come close to me. |
| Don't look at me. | Look at me. |
| I want to disappear. | I want to be here. |
| I'm not here. | I am here. |

Sit down comfortably together in a quiet place. Use these thought patterns to start with or listen for one the child may present herself.

Put the words *go away* in your right hand. As you repeat the phrase, let memories and associations arise. Talk about it. Keep building up the size and

Mereki is hyperopic only in her right eye. Here she Patches, bounces, and Paints White on her own eye chart.

color and weight of the energy Beach Ball in your right hand. Go to the opposite only when you have thoroughly explored the reality of this belief, only when you are totally satisfied that you have told the oceans and the dinosaurs, the sky, and everybody in the universe about it—that it is okay that everyone goes away because you can still love yourself a little bit when you are alone and rejected.

"Come close to me." It's okay that people are sometimes mean and hurtful. It's okay that sometimes they spit in your face and call you names. It's okay because you can still love yourself when they do this. You can still love yourself when you are hurting. Put "Come close to me" in your left-hand Beach Ball. Build it up to the stars, tell the Creator and the universe about it. Whisper it to the ants on the ground. Tell the baby birds in their nests. When you are satisfied with both your Beach Balls and they are somehow equal to one another, smoosh them together with a bang or a tiny sizzle. The baby birds are chirping happily and you can see clearly up close.

## Reversing Hyperopia with NVI

All the basic vision games in part two are helpful for hyperopia. However I'd like you to emphasize the following games:

- Cross-Crawl dancing to switch on the left side of the brain for your visual system (page 63).
- Movement. In general, hyperopes need lots of swings, free-form dancing, whole-body activities. Thoroughly absorb chapter 8. The Magic Nose Feather and the Bird Swing become a way of life. Refer to chapter 19 for setting up physical environments that encourage total body and eye coordination.
- Resting the eyes by Palming (page 106) and visualizing miniature worlds with lots of intricate details. A useful picture book for hyperopes ages three to ten is *The Bad-Tempered Ladybird* by Eric Carle. The print goes from small to large and back again while the grouchy ladybird (ladybug) meets aphids and a whale.
- The Magic Paintbrush Paints White (page 133) and Great White Glow (page 131) for reading large to small print.

### 👁 Shifting Images

Slide your Magic Nose Pencil from right to left on the following pictures.

The little person or animal will shift from side to side in the opposite direction you are moving. This restores superfast saccadic motions. When you close your eyes and shift the images in your imagination, the effect is fascinating.

Light a candle and place it directly in front of you. Opening and closing your eyes, sweep to the right and the left of the candle. Notice how the candle moves in the opposite direction. Sing this song:

THE CANDLE SWING

*Words and Melody by Helen M. Kennedy*

## The Ant Queen

Hyperopes need to imagine small close shapes in their mind. Use the following story while Palming. Edge and tickle the tiny images with your Magic Nose Feather.

Linda Sue loved ants. She spent hours lying on her tummy watching ants collect food. As an experiment, Linda Sue put half her cheese sandwich on an ant path. In twenty minutes the sandwich had been pulled apart into crumbs and carried away to the ant nest. One day while Linda Sue lay under a tree Palming, she decided to go and meet the Ant Queen.

Making herself tiny with shrink dust from the supermarket, Linda Sue knocked on the door of Anthill Seventeen. "Who's there?" demanded the ant who guarded the door. "It's me—Linda Sue, ant lover. I'm wearing my black hat and my black coat and my black socks and I'm wearing my black skydiving boots. Please let me come in. I want to visit your queen and see all her tiny treasures.

Grains of sand and bits of grass flew away from the entrance to the ants' underground home. A skinny hand waved Linda Sue inside the ant tunnel. "Follow me and be sure to tickle the earthworms with your Magic Nose Feather as you go past them. Otherwise they will feel insulted." Linda Sue followed the door-ant to a round room deep in the earth.

The Ant Queen, who was three times bigger than the humble door-ant, looked Linda Sue up and down with two emerald green eyes. In her hand the Ant Queen held a white paintbrush. She was painting ant eggs.

"Ten thousand and twenty-three. That's enough for today," sighed the Ant Queen. She put away her paintbrush, slopping a few drops of white paint on Linda Sue's skydiving boots. "What are those and what are you and what do you want?" The queen's green eyes glittered.

"Dear Queen, I'm an ant lover and I have come to *ohhh* and *ahhh* and edge with my Magic Nose Pencil all your tiny treasures. May I please?"

"At last, someone who understands art and beauty. Come here, my dear. Edge these cunning, rare, and priceless creatures." The Ant Queen opened a jade green box the size of your thumbnail. Inside the box three baby Christmas bugs slumbered on cherry red velvet. To Linda they looked like infant cockroaches that had been sprayed with metallic auto paint. But she didn't say anything. "Now I will show you something that no one up top should ever know about." "Up top" was what the ants called the surface of the earth. The Ant Queen tugged on a ring attached to a flat gray rock. The rock lifted; dust flew in all directions. A hundred gold eyes gleamed out of the dark hole. The Ant Queen scooped up one of the "eyes" and laid it in Linda Sue's hand as she whispered, "This is left over from our visit with the Spanish conquistadors." Linda Sue traced the round edges of a gold coin with her Magic Nose Pencil. She noticed faint lines scratched on its surface. She swept the coin with a delicate gold-colored Magic Nose Feather and read the words, "Love is everywhere. Alphonso Saltamontes 1492."

What other tiny objects could the Ant Queen show Linda Sue and Palming children in her treasure chamber? The first Ant Queen's baby rattle, the royal collection of matchbox cars, a fungus rock star in a jar, and microbes playing tennis.

Now it's your turn to imagine more tiny, miniature, miniscule, microscopic, wee things.

Daniel, Mereki, Soloman, and their mothers keep the Swinging Ball moving.

## 👁 The Swinging Ball

The Swinging Ball game brings forth saccadic movement and quick identification of shapes. It releases high spirits. Use a lightweight ball that won't hurt anyone who gets in the way. Styrofoam works well. Invite myopes into the game to help them lose their stare.

In fabric and craft shops you will find inexpensive white Styrofoam balls of various sizes. In Playcamps we use large fifteen-centimeter (six-inch) balls. Students paint them with acrylic paints in bright colors. Each ball is painted all over in a solid background color. When the background is dry, identifiable images are painted in contrasting colors, for example, stars, trees, cats, cars, or dots.

With pliers make a small eye on a length of stiff wire twenty centimeters (eight inches) long. Tie a one-meter- (three-foot-) long string to the wire eyelet. Pierce a channel through the middle of the foam ball with the wire. Pull the string through at the same time. Untie the string from the eyelet. Fasten a button or bead to the string so it cannot pull back through the ball. Remove the wire from the ball and hang the ball from a place where you can all lie in a circle underneath it, close enough to reach it with your hands and feet. Keep the ball swinging. As you bat the ball, follow it with your nose. Blink and breathe. See if you are able to edge a star or cat while the ball is traveling.

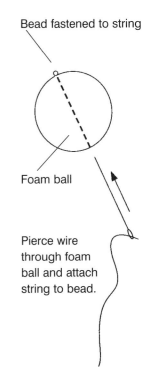

Bead fastened to string

Foam ball

Pierce wire through foam ball and attach string to bead.

### Timetable for Hyperopia Games

#### Birth to Two Years +

Do the Baby Eaglet Swing.
Bounce on the minitrampoline.
Have lots of crawling adventures.

#### Two to Ten Years +

Cross-Crawl dancing.
Palm for storytelling with small and close images.

#### Four to Ten Years +

The Swinging Ball.
Bird Swing.
Magic Nose Pencil.
Reading with the White Paintbrush.
Make and use your own black-and-white reading cards.
Resolve inner turmoil with the Melting Beach Balls.

Hyperopia is often accompanied by astigmatism and/or strabismus. If your child has a combination of these symptoms, the following chapters will help. On special days you would add games to iron out astigmatism and redirect eyes and brain toward fusion.

# 15

# Astigmatism

## What Is Astigmatism?

Astigmatism is usually a warp in the cornea at the front of the eye. It can also occur in the lens. The visual effect is akin to looking through an old window pane that has waves in it or in a carnival mirror.

There are two kinds of astigmatism, regular and irregular. The regular kind occurs at a particular angle and can be corrected with a cylindrical lens ground into glasses or healed with NVI. Irregular astigmatism is usually due to a disease condition or accident. It cannot be satisfactorily corrected by glasses.

A distorted cornea creates astigmatism.

### How Astigmatism Feels and Looks

Astigmatism causes visual blur and tired eyes at all distances. Even a slight amount can result in aching, scratchy eyes after reading for five minutes. Distortion in the distance can be unnoticeable until you have to read a street sign. If the warp is vertical, all the upright letters, such as *E, P, B, T,* and *L,* will be blurred posts. If you have astigmatism at 60 degrees, the *Z* in *Zebra* will be blurred.

A cylindrical lens corrects for astigmatism.

## The Cause of Astigmatism

In ophthalmic literature, astigmatism is blamed on the upper eyelid pressing on the cornea. Dr. Duke-Elder states that 68 percent of children at the age of four and 95 percent at the age of seven have this kind of astigmatism. When the child grows older, pressure astigmatism tends to disappear or reverse itself into the opposite angle.

Sixty-degree astigmatism will do this to a Z.

Normal vision, no astigmatism

This figure shows horizontal astigmatism. It is corrected by a cylindrical lens at axis 180 degrees.

Here oblique astigmatism blurs everything at 45 degrees. It is corrected by a cylindrical lens at 45 degrees.

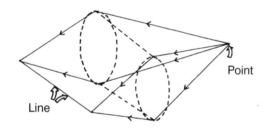

A cylindrical lens focuses a line to a point.

You can produce astigmatism easily for yourself right now by pressing your finger against your eyelid or "by the action of the extra-ocular muscles," as Duke-Elder writes. The extraocular muscles are those six big muscles (page 74) that rotate and move the eyeball in all directions. Could a pair of muscles be holding tight?

A cylindrical lens is placed in glasses to compensate for astigmatism in the optical system of the eyes.

## How Correction Is Determined

Optometrists and ophthalmologists employ both mechanical and subjective means of determining the amount and angle of astigmatism correction. If a child is old enough to respond adequately, the doctor will try with the best of intentions to come up with an accurate prescription by placing a lens and a letter in front of the child's eyes. The question is asked, "Is this better or is this better?" as the lenses are changed. As an astigmatic child, I remember being confused and stressed by this questioning. I perspired in my effort to give that nice man the right answer.

# It Appears and Disappears

Astigmatism distortion in the eyes and in the visual field can be here at one o'clock and gone at two o'clock. I had challenged my students many times in teacher training courses with this statement. Finally a certified teacher in Munich paid her money and visited three different optometrists in one afternoon. Sure enough, she came home with three different prescriptions. The amount of astigmatism changes. The angle shifts. If you yourself have old prescriptions for astigmatism in your drawer, take a look. Notice if strength and direction have changed.

A child's eyes will continually attempt to please a correction ground into his lenses. Doing the activities in this chapter will help smooth away astigmatism warp. If your child puts glasses back on with correction for astigmatism in them, his progress is wiped out.

If members of the optical industry find a trace of astigmatism during an eye exam, most of them will insist on putting correction for it into the child's glasses. Their motives are impeccable: "He will get headaches and severe eyestrain if we do not correct for astigmatism." They have the best of intentions and don't want anyone to suffer the pain of uncorrected astigmatism.

I speak from acute personal experience. My last pair of fully corrected lenses had five diopters of astigmatism correction for my right eye and two diopters for my left. Conscientious optometrists and medical doctors drew careful diagrams for me of the eyeball, sympathized with my inevitable reading distress, and insisted on a correction for astigmatism. I insisted back. In my first pair of T-Glasses the astigmatism was cut by half to two and one-half diopters for my right eye. It was taken out completely on the left side.

In the guidelines for T-Glasses, I say, "Take out all astigmatism correction if possible." In my case the warp on my right cornea was too great to immediately cut out all astigmatism correction. I needed some of it to see 6/12 (20/40) through my driving glasses. Astigmatism correction may have to be juggled with myopic or hyperopic correction. You need an extremely cooperative practitioner who understands that you will be playing "erase astigmatism" games with your child. If your son needs to see the board at school, it may be necessary to leave some astigmatism correction in his lenses; but I stipulate, with caution: if he has less than one diopter, leave it out.

# An Astigmatism Prescription

A prescription for astigmatism only, in one eye only, should look like the illustration below. The word *axis* designates the angle of astigmatism. The cylindrical lens is ground in the glasses at the angle determined by an optometrist or ophthalmologist

Think about geometry. For example, if the axis number is 45, then a cylindrical lens is placed at 45 degrees, as you see on the figure below right.

*Note:* The word *sphere* in the prescription example refers to a correction for either myopia (a minus "-" will appear before the number of diopters) or hyperopia (a plus "+" will appear before the number of diopters). Astigmatism usually occurs in combination with myopia or hyperopia, rarely all by itself.

|  | SPH (sphere) | CYL (cylinder) | AXIS |
|---|---|---|---|
| **Right Eye** |  | -1 | x15 |
| **Left Eye** |  |  |  |

# Erase Astigmatism with NVI

Emphasize switching on the whole brain with Cross-Crawl dancing. Do Bird Swings. Using the Great White Glow and Magic Paintbrush when reading will minimize fatigue and blur.

The following games for astigmatism can be played in two ways. Sweeping along every angle will help saccadic movement and eye mobility in general. The game can be made more specific if you know the angle of astigmatism. You can then spend most of your time sweeping your Magic Nose Feather or Magic Paintbrush along that angle.

The angle and amount of astigmatism could be different in each eye. In this case, you can separate the eyes by using a Pirate Patch (see page 182).

### Zoo Train

Guide your child through the following activity.

With your Magic Nose Feather swing and sweep on the vertical part of the railway track for a few seconds.

Close your eyes and do exactly the same movement, keeping the image of the railway track in your mind.

Northeast

Zoo Train

Southwest

Open your eyes again, sweeping up and down the track. Repeat the same process with the horizontal railway track.

Do the same three-step process with the northeast and southwest tracks. Imagine that a train engine takes off around the figure-eight track. Give it a color. Pink with green smoke? Good. Close your eyes and imagine it traveling around the whole track. Open again. After the train makes three complete revolutions around the track, it picks up a freight car. The freight car is also pink. It contains a yawning lion. Follow the train around the track with engine and one lion car, eyes open, eyes closed. Attach another car. The second car—pink, of course—contains a giraffe. You can see its long neck sticking out. Around and around we go, eyes open for a while, then closed. You can add as many cars and animals as you like. This becomes a memory game. For advanced players, change the colors of the cars. Photocopy the Zoo Train or draw your own version.

Your goal is to loosen up external eye muscles that guide the eyes along the designated angle. This is done with right-brain imagery and movement along that angle. It helps to make your own visual games, both on paper and in the landscape.

## Birds on a Wire Game

Take a ruler and draw a straight black line on paper at the angle of astigmatism shown on the prescription. Your child then draws birds on the "wire." After the birds are drawn, he then slides up and down or back and forth on that line with his eyes open for a few seconds. Follow by imagining the Birds on a Wire with eyes closed for a few seconds, then again with eyes open. (Do not be terribly precise about the angle, as it is probably wriggling around anyway.) Make sure

Birds on a wire at 135 degrees

An astigmatism turtle for vertical and horizontal astigmatism

your child keeps his head level when sweeping along the wire so his eyes are saccadically vibrating at the appropriate angle. You can vary this game by asking your child for his favorite theme: draw a series of dinosaurs marching along the wire, cars, coins, or soccer balls. Draw balloons, lollipops, or birds flying, animals, flowers, spiderwebs, spaceships, or goldfish. Do it on paper, then imagine your goldfish are swimming on the wall, then across the sky.

After swinging and sweeping along friendly images on paper, walls, and skies, sing this song. Follow along all the lines you can find with your Magic Nose Pencil.

Plants and animals at 180 degrees

Goldfish at 45 degrees

# LINES, STRAIGHT LINES

*Music – Traditional, Words by NVI Teacher Dede Callichy*

Lines, straight lines, Lines, straight lines. See how they run,

See how they run! From top to bot-tom and side to side,

All are straight, some nar-row some wide. Have you seen such a won-der-ful sight in your life as

lines, straight lines?

# What Astigmatism Feels Like Inside

Astigmatic eyes ache. It is seeing at the emotional level of pain. The unconscious thought is "It hurts to see." This is evidenced by an indirect response in eye muscles, either the large outside muscles pulling across the cornea or the ciliary muscle tugging on the lens of the eye.

Astigmatism results in painful seeing at all distances. Reading makes sandpaper eyes. When looking into the distance, there is a sensation of displacement. Even though the hills and buildings are upright, there's a warped feeling inside the mind.

Adult NVI students with a lot of astigmatism stopped using correction so they could explore painful sensations previously blocked by their glasses. Sometimes they sat still, gazing steadily at a black line held at their angle of astigmatism. During this exercise a woman in Germany with vertical astigmatism recalled being left behind in her baby bed when everyone else ran to the bomb shelters. Tobias Mosner, an NVI instructor, wrote down these thoughts that arose for him:

> I don't belong in this world.
> I don't trust myself.
> I don't trust where I take myself with my own ideas.
> The astigmatism shift keeps me away from myself.
> Everything I do is wrong. Everyone else is right.

## Emotional Healing for Astigmatism

Four main issues emerge as mental and emotional partners to astigmatism:

| | |
|---|---|
| It hurts to see. | Seeing feels good. |
| I hate myself. | I love myself. |
| I mistrust myself. | Everything I do is valid. |
| I don't belong here. | I'm in the right place. |

There are children who cannot abide making a mistake or getting anything less than an A on their schoolwork. Humiliation and internal burning shame that are covered up with a blanket or shoved into a drawer can become a lifelong reaction. To ease this hidden stress, we must teach these children that love is still here for people who fail. This may be a great challenge if your child is attending school and being rewarded for perfect performance. The school system rewards their stress mechanism with accolades.

Myopes are seeking approval and love from outside themselves. If a young myope also has astigmatism, you have a deluxe recipe for denial of life. Don't be too shocked when opening a box of suppressed emotions to hear a voice say, "I want to die." The death wish pattern affects the kidney meridian, whose affirmation is "I love being alive." In Chinese medicine, eye disturbances are linked to the kidney meridian.

Let's deal first with the theme "I hate myself." It may be difficult to conceive that small children are already judging and rejecting themselves. Yet anyone who has worked with a child perfectionist or a child with learning difficulties knows that this theme of self-disapproval is constantly active, even at home and on the playground.

## Use the Melting Beach Balls

Put "I hate myself" in your right hand (see Melting Beach Balls, page 119). Make it into an energy ball with color and weight. Build it up while you repeat the words "I hate myself." Is it okay to hate yourself?

It's okay to hate myself, yes.

Is it okay to bring it out and say it out loud, even yell it to the treetops until it is somehow funny?

Next you ask for the opposite. Your child may have a different answer from "I love myself." Go with the child's truth.

"I love myself; I love myself." Feel how the sound of these words vibrates in your body. If it's not true yet, then go right back to the opposite, until you can return and enjoy "I love myself."

Okay. Under all circumstances, I can love myself, even when I don't know the answer to the math problem; even when I say something stupid; even when I hurt someone else's feelings and need to apologize. It's okay to hate and to love myself.

Bring both Beach Balls together like party balloons, like colored foam, like . . . well, you tell me. . . .

# Other Therapies

Astigmatism can be mechanically related to displaced skull bones: Contrary to popular belief, skull bones never completely fuse together. The eye socket is constructed of several moveable bones. These bones encasing the eyes and optic nerves can be manually adjusted. In children the skull is extremely flexible. Osteopathic textbooks show photographs of children's heads that had been distorted by difficult births: by forceps or suction delivery. In many cases adjustment of the skull bones resulted in improved sight as astigmatism disappeared. Some chiropractors are trained to perform adjustments to the skull. Look for an osteopath or chiropractor who does craniopathy.

# 16

# Strabismus and Lazy Eyes

## What Is Strabismus?

An eye muscle that does not release or relax fully can hold an eye in a fixed position, away from the line of sight. This condition is called strabismus, or squint, depending on how severe the turn may be. In this chapter I will use the word *strabismus* interchangeably with "turned eye."

The muscles of a turned eye are either not receiving correct messages from the brain or, if the message does come through, may be unable to respond because the bone to which they are attached is tilted within the skull. When the brain says look straight ahead, or left or right, the pair of eye muscles that turn the eyes in the desired direction do not respond properly. One muscle remains cramped, and its partner refuses to contract.

There is usually nothing wrong with the eyeball itself, unless squint has been started by a disease process. A turned eye can become a "lazy eye" if the message from that eye is not used by the visual brain in the process of seeing.

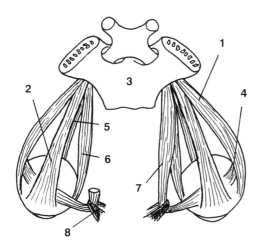

1  **Lateral rectus**
2  **Superior rectus**
3  **Sphenoid bone**
4  **Inferior oblique muscle**
5  **Inferior rectus**
6  **Medial rectus**
7  **Superior oblique muscle**
8  **Trochlea; the superior oblique muscle slides through this pulley**

Eye Muscles are directed from the brain and are attached to skull bones.

Exotropia means the eye turns outward (walleyed). The eye diverges.

Esotropia means the eye turns inward (cross-eyed). The eye converges.

This is what turned eyes look like from outside:

*Alternating squint* means the child looks first with one eye, then with the other. The "switched-off" eye usually goes inward.

Misalignment of eyes can occur in other directions as well. Even a slight deviation from ideal coordination results in fatigue and disturbance of some brain functions.

A turned eye signifies unbalanced brain activity. Human eyes are designed to work together, simultaneously pointing toward and saccadically vibrating around the same point in space. The organism must use 500 percent of body energy, instead of the usual 25 percent allocated to vision, to overcome misalignment. Ultimately, the brain decides to turn off the message from one eye, conserving energy for other duties. A lazy eye results. The official term for lazy eye is *amblyopia ex anopsia*. If remedial action of some kind is taken, amblyopia can be avoided or reversed.

## Why Eyes Turn

Medical information given to parents describes the crooked tree but not its roots. In *The Well Baby Book*, Dr. Samuels explains, "The eyes are not properly aligned due to unequal strength and faulty balance in the muscles surrounding the eye." The next question hangs in the air: "What causes unequal strength and muscular imbalance?"

Searching for the root cause of strabismus led me to dig deeper, via medical textbooks and phone calls to osteopaths and behavioral optometrists.

Cameron Dawson, of Dawson Technologies in Victoria, Australia, teaches therapists to correct strabismus by gentle manipulation of the cranial bones. Eye muscles attach to skull bones. "In the majority of cases, turned eyes result from the bones of the skull not being in the correct position."

Behavioral optometrists sometimes blame turned eyes on environmental interferences during the binocular development stage. Richard Kavner, O.D., in his book *Your Child's Vision*, says head injuries from forceps deliveries can be a cause. But he feels that most often there is a disturbance of the neural control centers in the brain.

Dr. Bates would say that eyes are turning because the child is making an effort to see. When his small patients relaxed their minds and eyes, their eyes straightened.

Parents have a number of options to consider.

## The Medical Response

Medical textbooks do not address in any depth emotional, mental, environmental, or historical (birth trauma) factors in squint. Therefore medically trained doctors will recommend a purely physical approach, which, according to Duke-Elder, is a surgical plaster over the straight eye day and night for three months. "The defective eye is thus coerced into activity." The child must be checked by the doctor during this period "since the deviation sometimes becomes transferred to the occluded (covered) eye and the vision in it may deteriorate."

*Atropine* drops may be given to the parents to place in the child's good eye. With atropine, distance vision becomes blurred and near vision becomes impossible. Atropine is a drug that affects the autonomic nervous system.

From *Mim's Manual:* "Atropine sulphate is widely used in ophthalmology as a powerful mydriatic and cycloplegic. Dilation of the pupil occurs within half an hour of its local application and lasts for a week or so. Atropine is used both pre-operatively and post-operatively in many types of intraocular surgery. It is also used in refractive work with children."

In Australia, atropine sulfate is listed as an S4 medicinal poison. The regulations regarding S4 poisons vary somewhat from state to state. For Western Australia we read:

S4 to be labeled Caution, supply without prescription illegal: keep out of reach of children. Supply restricted to prescription or authorized person with an allowance for some emergency supply for continuation of human therapy. Prescription to be cancelled unless repeated. Order validity 12 months. Advertising not permitted except in bona fide professional journals. Records of prescriptions dispensed to be maintained.

Duke-Elder states:

> The results of such treatment are very varying. If the eye were amblyopic (and turning) before treatment commenced, the good eye would be occluded for a month, and if no improvement occurs a further month may be tried. If this too proves fruitless, all hope of ultimate functional utility may be abandoned. If better vision can be elicited, occlusion should be continued. Provided the case is carefully supervised, there need be no hesitation in continuing this for considerable periods of time, as long as any improvement is obtained.

At this point the surgeon may decide on *orthoptic* treatment: visual training for binocular vision. If orthoptic training does not work, the next step is surgically clipping the overtight muscle or resetting its attachment to the eyeball. This is done under general anesthesia.

Language is a powerful tool. It can become a cattle prod when used by authority figures. If you feel threatened or intimidated by medical jargon or emotionally loaded words, admit it. This will allow you to avoid being goaded into actions you feel in your heart are wrong. *Blind* is a particularly frightening term. "Your child will go blind in that eye if she does not have an operation now." Let's examine this message under a magnifying glass.

The word *blind* used in this context signifies amblyopia. The eye is not blind in the usual sense. In fact if the "good eye" were destroyed, the turning eye would come back onstage. In most cases the turned eye is physically healthy. This use of the word *blind* is therefore highly misleading. Notice its effect in your nervous system and hesitate twice before making a decision out of panic.

What about the time pressure? If you wait any longer your child will go *blind*. Pause at least long enough to consult with three unconnected medical specialists and with behavioral optometrists who work directly with strabismus. David Evian, O.D., who runs a clinic in Sydney, Australia, for strabismus training, asserts, "For every theory there is a countertheory."

The "closed window" theory says that if overtight muscles are not operated upon during a certain time in the child's brain development, it will be too late: the window slams shut. Does the window open and close between four and six months, between birth and age five, between ages four and ten? Or does it never close? The professionals have varying opinions:

- *You must operate on this baby with a turned eye before it is six months old.* From studies covering the eyes of chicks and kittens, it has been found that after this stage the cells in the visual cortex will no longer respond and the child will never get fusion. Operate now.

- *Children with squint must be operated on before the age of seven.* After that they will not get fusion, nor will they be able to speak a foreign language without an accent, as the appropriate cells in the brain will not be willing to learn a new pattern.
- *This cross-eyed child must be operated on before the age of ten.* After that the organism is too set in its ways.

Imagine a conference where ophthalmologists, perception psychologists, neurologists, pediatricians, behavioral optometrists, osteopaths, and chiropractors got together to discuss the "closed window" theory. Fur would fly.

# Behavioral Optometrists Train Turned Eyes

The goal of ophthalmic surgery and orthoptics is fused binocular vision. Everyone doing vision training has this same goal, including optometrists and NVI teachers.

Behavioral optometrists use visual training with optical devices rather than surgery and drugs or surgery plus orthoptics. There are ten to twenty clinics in Australia where full training services are offered for children on a weekly basis. I spoke with Graeme Thompson, representative of the ACBO, the Australasian College of Behavioral Optometrists, in Sydney. He said, "A lot of surgery is done, but it is a cosmetic success. The eyes are straight, but the function is still strabismic. You can't gauge success by the appearance of the eyes."

Dr. Richard Kavner states the case more strongly: "A parent who seeks advice about a child's turned eye is frequently told that the only thing to do is to have ocular surgery. Not only is this advice incorrect and misleading, it can be dangerous in ways we hadn't thought of before. In fact, relatively few cases of strabismus are due to faulty muscles. Surgery may therefore be entirely unjustified in many cases."

Every operation using anesthesia carries risk.

By 1978 eleven independent surveys assessing the success rate of orthoptics for strabismus had been made. The results varied from 34.2 percent to 92.7 percent. This data came from both optometric and ophthalmic sources. The two optometrists who collated the surveys concluded, "Although the ophthalmological-orthoptist strabismus cure rates of 56 percent achieving high level functional cures and 67 percent achieving cosmetic success are impressive figures, the optometric studies show a high level functional cure rate of 76 percent and almost 86 percent cosmetic success." A "functional cure" means the children are achieving fusion. "Cosmetic success" tells you the eyes are straight but the messages from the two eyes are not being used simultaneously by the visual brain.

# Cranial Adjustment

For this book Cameron Dawson writes:

Conventional anatomy teaches that the bones of the skull are separate at birth and become one solid static cranial structure in adult life. The baby's head needs to be very flexible at birth to fold the cranial plates gently, allowing access into the world through the birth canal. Every mother in the Western world is made aware of the fact that the open areas between the cranial plates, the fontanels, are to be avoided to limit any damage to the baby's brain. This misinformation is the root cause of the problems of strabismus and learning difficulties. What mother indeed is going to allow any untoward pressure to her beautiful new baby's head, but this inhibits her taking the natural action that every other mammal mother takes in caressing by hand or tongue the head of the newborn. This attention by the mother is a natural instinct and places cranial plates back into correct position after they've been misaligned through the birth process. Fortunately statistics show that two out of three babies achieve the correct alignment of the head bones by chance and there is no further problem. It is the other 30-odd percent where problems arise.

Balinese people follow an ancient practice derived from their Polynesian and Indian heritage. Babies are massaged at birth, both body and head, for a moon and two days. The mother is taught this technique by her mother-in-law. Bodily massage continues in another form throughout the child's lifetime.

In America, the home of cranial osteopathy, the skulls of newborns are checked by osteopathic physicians for birth trauma. Slight or gross damage to the skull can cause constant unexplained crying, breathing disorders, frequent infections, learning problems, astigmatism, and strabismus. Like the Point Holding described in chapter 6, remedial treatment is light, rhythmic, and sustained until a change is detected.

In NVI seminars adults who had numerous operations as children, and whose eyes still turned, were able to obtain fusion. This was accomplished with switching on the whole brain, with directional fusion games, and with Emotional Healing. Every one of these people cried with joy when they looked in the mirror at two straight eyes, eyes that were ready to play fusion games. A man in Virginia, who had spent twenty years trying to get fusion, said orthoptists had thrown him out as a hopeless case. I suggested he remember a scene from his childhood, instead of trying to fuse with his left brain. He was instantly successful. A letter six months later reported that he still had fusion.

## Your Options

- *Wait and see; do nothing.* This is not my style, but I honor anyone's right to do this. A woman once said to me that she had healed her eyesight through prayer. I honor that approach too.
- *Take your child immediately to an ophthalmologist for a thorough exam, diagnosis, and recommended medical treatment.* I think it is a good idea to get an expert diagnosis. However, if seeking treatment, I would certainly roam far and wide to find a person and a clinic where the treatment process does not traumatize the child. Surgical treatment is more readily available than anything else, but it leaves a trail of shattered and frightened children who sometimes refuse any kind of help thereafter—even if it is NVI fun and games mildly presented under a tree. When they hear the words *eyes, fusion, doctor, clinic,* some of these children freeze up or disappear out the door.
- *Seek examination and treatment with vision training from a behavioral optometrist.* Behavioral optometrists are trained to thoroughly examine eyes and prescribe glasses and/or visual training for children with strabismus. Seek out someone who has an empathetic assistant who will serve as teacher and friend to the child. These sessions usually run for an hour once a week.
- *Search for and use natural therapies.* Oh, for a Balinese mother-in-law, a skilled cranial osteopath, or even a chiropractor trained in cranial adjustments! You may have to search high and low, or travel, but such rare birds do exist. In the meantime, use the vision games and the resources in this book.

- *Find yourself an NVI teacher or train to become one yourself* (see page 240). Please note that NVI is not a substitute for examination and diagnosis of eyes, as we are not trained to do either of these. We are, however, prepared and educated to play vision games and do Emotional Healing with children in a human, informal fashion that can be used in conjunction with any of the approaches given above, except the first one.

# Straighten Turned Eyes with NVI

The most important thing to remember when playing Natural Vision Improvement games with turning eyes is the concept of phoria. *Phoria* is Latin for "tendency." It is used in the optical industry to designate the tendency of the line of vision to deviate from normal.

## Favoring the Phoria

Favoring the phoria means inviting (rather than coercing) the turning eye to move in the desired direction. For example, if the right eye wants to stick to the nose, then we wish to entice (not force) the right eye to look in an outward direction. Usually people say the eye must be made to work. Don't work an eye, muscle, or brain that is already under stress. Let the eye and its muscles relax and play along with the child they belong to.

Favoring the phoria with ducky

### Principles to Remember for Favoring the Phoria

Use the following ideas and vision games to coax and invite turned eyes in the direction they need to go.

#### Eyes are attracted to light and movement with
penlights
a ball on a string
candles
wind chimes
glitter
bells and windmills

## Eyes are attracted to color and contrast

Use complementary colors when making Tromboning Paddles (page 177):

black and white
blue and orange
red and green
yellow and violet

Contrary to assumption, tiny children do have long attention spans. When the entertainment is paced to the child's level and kept simple, she will extend the game and ask for repetition. Carina at nine months pulled a pair of underpants on and off her head ninety-seven times. Aerro at nineteen months performed an acrobatic somersault over my body twelve times in succession, applauding himself after each roll.

Gently covering the straight eye, talk to the turning eye.

## Games for Babies with Turned Eyes

### Birth to One Year +

Make eating into a phoria game with the Flying Spoon. Get the baby's attention with delicious food on a spoon. Bring the spoon toward her from the appropriate side. It can do some aeronautical tricks before it lands in her mouth.

Hang her batting mobiles so that the kicking foot attracts her eye in the desired direction.

Play tug-of-war. Lay baby on the floor. Let her tug on the towels.

Touch draws the attention of the eyes. If something crawls across your skin while you are lying outdoors under a tree, you jerk to attention and send your eyes in that direction, to identify the crawler as friend or foe. Should you kiss it or swat it?

Most people instinctively use their fingers to draw an infant's attention. Notice from which direction you do this with a baby whose eye turns and sticks. Before age three months the child's eye probably won't turn in the direction of a tickle, but we are investing in later habits, and after three months your cooing and tickling will begin to induce attention and eye movement in the desired direction. The next song will help.

## WHERE IS THAT TICKLE

*Words and Music by Donald Woodward*

Where is that tic-kle? That tic-kle, ic-kle, ic-kle?
Look where I tic-kle. I tic-kle, ic-kle, ic-kle.

Where is that tic-kle ic-kle-ee?
Look where I tic-kle ic-kle-ee.

Where is that tic-kle? That tic-kle, ic-kle, ic-kle,
Look where I tic-kle. I tic-kle, ic-kle, ic-kle.

Where is that tic-kle go-ing to be?
Look where I tic-kle, ic-kle-ee.

## Directional Tromboning

Tromboning is the simple action of moving an interesting object near and far, close to the eye and away. It induces accommodation activity in the lens and activates extrinsic muscles. Use Tromboning to coax, entice, or seduce a reluctant eye in the direction you'd like it to go. Anything can be tromboned: a favorite doll, a master of the universe, a plastic dinosaur, a flashy ring, a pink petunia, a piece of toast. A deck of playing cards could be used, or purchased card games such as Rummy or Old Maid.

### Three Months to One Year

Covering the child's straight or stronger eye with one hand, slowly bring a toy toward and away from her. I discovered that if I sing or murmur while doing this, the baby looks at my mouth instead of the object. When choosing a toy for Directional Tromboning, use objects that twinkle or make a noise.

After the child is four months old, make sure the object is mouthable. She will grab it for spatial exploration with her tongue.

### Two to Ten Years +

Make your own paddles: A paddle is cut out of stiff cardboard in a shape that is easy to hold on to while moving it to and from the eye.

A Tromboning paddle

For example, let us make an animal-sticker paddle. Cut your piece of cardboard in the shape shown. Then cover it with animal stickers or cut-out animals from magazines. I suggest both parent and child have a paddle. Tromboning keeps parents from ever needing reading glasses. Younger children can sit on your lap. Your child may allow you to cover her straight eye for a minute while she watches her paddle come near and far. Older children will hold their own paddles. After age six your child's paddle collection can sit on her desk or hang from the bedpost.

When tromboning, call out the name of an animal—for example, "kitty cat." Add the sound: *meow*. Cow: *mooooo*. Make paddles with colored circles or a combination of geometric figures; construct favorite-theme paddles. If your child likes cars, buy a car magazine and attack it with scissors. As you trombone with the paddle, either for the child or when she does it for herself, you still want to be favoring the phoria each time.

If right eye goes out, the paddle moves across your body's midline and outward to the left.

If left eye goes out, the paddle moves across your body's midline and outward to the right.

If left eye goes in, the paddle moves away from your body's midline toward the left.

If right eye goes in, the paddle moves away from your body's midline toward the right.

For an eye that drifts outward, cover the other eye and hold the paddle in front of you. Trombone the paddle in and out, crossing the midline of your body to draw the eye toward your nose (figures A and B).

Hum, croon, drone, tone, tiddle a ditty as you trombone. This switches on the right side of the brain. The paddle pictures will in turn attract the turning eye back onstage.

For an eye that pulls too far inward, the moving paddle is used to escort the eye in an outward direction (figures C and D).

Covering the opposite eye with the palm of the hand, trombone the paddle from the nose outward, away from the midline of your (the child's) body.

## "Photographing" the Light

Instructions in this section are addressed to the adult who will guide the child.

### Six to Ten Years +

You and your child should stand with your backs to a light source such as a standing lamp. Turn the lamp so the bulb is visible. Make sure the lamp is incandescent. Never use a suntanning bulb. The sun could be used as a light source also, in the morning or late afternoon, as you will be moving across it only briefly.

Cover the straight eye with the palm of your hand. Both eyes remain open. Keeping your feet in the same spot, do a swing with your whole body around to the light source. Circle the light once, then close both eyes and let your body swing back to its original position. After doing this a few times, you will notice that the afterimage of the lightbulb on your eyelid has moved in the direction you want your turned eye to go. *Adults:* Please experiment with this until you get it right yourself, then teach it to your child.

## Phoria Ball Games

Every child loves a ball. Her first one may be a soft, chewy type. Then come the ones that jingle as they roll. The bouncy, big ones are hot stuff to throw for toddlers. Then you start to play catch. Please make dropping the ball part of the game. No Little League competition here. Collect balls and keep them in a box or basket for phoria play at first and later to play with while Patching.

## Timetable for Phoria Ball Games

### Four Months to One Year +

Hide a ball and have it emerge from a surprising place.
Swing a foam ball decorated wildly with glitz and glitter
on an elastic string.

### One to Five Years +

Roll the ball all over your body while laughing and
massaging.
Take all the round fruit out of a fruit bowl and roll it to your child.
Bounce a ball on the ground on the side favoring the phoria.
Call your child's name and send the ball to her.

If her left eye goes
in, roll the ball to her
left side.

### Five to Ten Years +

Play soccer with your child; as goalkeeper, always kick the ball to the
side favoring the phoria.
Play table tennis and hit the ball to the side that favors the phoria.
Put a foam ball in paint and roll it on paper.
Play with glass marbles, placing the holes or goals on the side favoring
the phoria.
Play catch with a ball. Pretend it is a hot potato.
Buy a colored beach ball to throw on the side favoring the phoria.
Call out the colors.
Throw a ball against a wall; turn around before it comes down to the
side where the turned eye has to look first.
Always talk to each other favoring the phoria.

## 👁 Who's That in the Mirror?

### Four Months to Two Years

While your child is still light enough, hold her in front of you—both facing
the same way. Stand with your backs to a mirror. Swivel your bodies toward
the mirror, keeping your feet facing forward. Exclaim and crow when you
see your reflections. "Who's that in the mirror?" "Why, it's Joanie!"

If you are turning in the correct direction for favoring the phoria, Joanie's inward turning eye will be stimulated to move outward by the happy sight of herself. If Joanie's eye is turning outward, you will have to swing across your midline so the turned eye is coaxed toward her nose. Sing this song.

## THE MIRROR SONG

*Words and Melody by Helen M. Kennedy*

Peek and close,_____ Peek and close,_____
Peek and close and then,_____
Peek and close,_____ Peek and close,_____
Peek and close a - gain._____

## The Windmill Swing

If your right eye is going inward, stand erect with your feet planted on the ground. Cover your left eye with your left hand. Pretend you right arm is a windmill. Swing it up and back, around and around. Follow your swinging hand with your right eye. In your hand you might like to hold an imaginary owl that has come to have a ride on the windmill.

If your left eye wanders inward, cover your right eye with your right hand. Pretend your left arm is a windmill. Swing it up and back, around and around. Follow your swinging hand with your left eye. Perhaps a giant orange-and-black monarch butterfly would like to take a ride on your fingertip.

"The Windmill Song" was written by Helen Kennedy. When she passed away in Los Angeles, her family gifted all her Corbett teaching materials to me. Helen had taught hundreds of children to see clearly with straight eyes.

Felicity shows you how to do the Windmill Swing for a right eye that goes in.

This is the movement if your left eye goes in.

Aerro the Pirate

## Pirate Patching

Patching the straight eye gives the turning eye a chance to come onstage by itself for a time. The visual brain that belongs to the unpatched eye will be stimulated. Obtain your eye patches from drugstores, or order bright-colored ones from us by mail order.

Medical patching is often not effective because the child is totally miserable. This memory lingers in the nervous system. The joy of interacting with others, music, and games should be connected with patching, as opposed to the trauma, poison, and pain of other methods. Misery switches off the right brain and keeps it off. This inhibits brain integration, a prerequisite for fused eyes. The brain needs an invitation to help eye muscles relax and vibrate, give and take. Coercion is 99 percent ineffective and counterproductive in any learning process. A new language is best learned while listening to Mozart, switching on both sides of the brain. A new visual habit is best instilled with right-brain levity.

### Games to Play When Pirating

Dale the pirate

Cross-Crawl dancing (page 63)
Bird Swing (page 80)
Near-Far Swing (page 82)
Circle and count (page 94)
The Candle Swing (page 153)
Look into a crystal ball or through a quartz crystal while lying on your
     back.
Do matching games with cards and pictures.
Play catch and run after balls.
Read a picture book. Favoring the phoria, edge the pictures with your
     Magic Nose Pencil.
Make cookies, salads, sandwiches—pirate food.
With older children, play marbles or tiddlywinks, slot car racing, video
     games and Nintendo. Do role-playing games with Cyclops, the one-
     eyed monster. Do Cross-Crawl dancing of course. Play "I spy" and "I
     went to visit my auntie in Alaska."
"Search and find" picture books are popular. Martin Handlord's *Where's
     Wally?* books and posters have traveled around the globe. *Where's
     Wendy?* designed by Anthony Tallarico, is a less violent version of a
     finding game. An exciting picture riddle book with photographic

realism is *I Spy Fantasy: A Book of Picture Riddles* by Walter Wick and
Jean Marzollo. For the older children, I recommend *For Eagle Eyes
Only* and *Ultimaze* by Rolf Heinmann.

Make this song a family heirloom.

Heave ho, me hearties!

Decorate your eye patches. Do them up in football team colors using fabric paints. Take a scarf and patch all the stuffed toys in the house. Have a collection of hats with patches attached. Sew sequins, ribbons, fabric patches to eye patches. Draw family patching portraits.

## Emotional Healing for Strabismus

In human culture, fairy tales, and schoolyards, any person with a turned eye is the wicked stepsister, the ugly duckling.

The vast majority of children with turned eyes are also hyperopic. This group of people have the challenge of playing the misfits in the school system. They are most often designated as the ones with "learning difficulties." The school system consists of round holes. Hyperopic cross-eyed children are square pegs. They are often dealing with thought patterns that make them outcasts, failures, and rejects.

Wilhelm Reich believed that hyperopes are suppressing anger. When their feelings boil over, havoc results. This is a "difficult child." It is far easier for adults to tolerate an anxious-to-please myopic child than a turbulent, noisy, bull-in-the-china-shop hyperope. To conformist neurotic myopes, these rowdies may appear psychotic.

On one level, I feel that cross-eyed hyperopic children are one notch healthier than the myopes. Their aliveness is more evident. Reich enjoyed his psychotic patients. They had a unique, direct insight into reality, even if their behavior was unacceptable to society. Cross-eyed children have to work very hard to make themselves acceptable. First, I suggest they be encouraged to express and resolve their anger. Second, they need to find a way to esteem and nurture their novel perceptions.

- Sit down or, better yet, dance wildly with this child while singing out these thought patterns:

  I'm mad.
  I'm a failure.
  I'm wild and dangerous.
  I'm . . .

- Use Melting Beach Balls (page 119).

Some word patterns I've heard from cross-eyed children:

| | |
|---|---|
| I'm ugly. | I'm beautiful. |
| I'm crooked. | I'm straight. |
| I don't fit in here. | This is my place. |

The nasty stepsister with a cast in her eye in fairy tales is an archetype representing the ugly side of ourselves that we all want to reject. Strabismic children, consciously or unconsciously, have the special task of transmuting this rejected side of humanity. This is true even if yours is the cutest cross-eyed child in the world. It is a unique opportunity for us all to deal with the part of us that we condemn. Loving ourselves when we are ugly and when we are beautiful is the key.

Using the Beach Balls, place "I'm ugly" in one hand. Give your Beach Ball a color. Make it huge. Yell "I'm ugly" to the sky or whisper it to the Easter bunny. Express it until you are satisfied with the size, weight, and color of your "I'm ugly" Beach Ball.

Then ask, "What is the opposite of ugly?" Some children may have a different expression. If it is "I'm cute," put "I'm cute," or "I'm handsome," in the opposite hand. Expand the phrase with sound and color into a Beach Ball that

**THE CROSS-EYED MONSTER**

*Music – Tradtional, Words by Janet Goodrich*

I'm a lit-tle mon-ster, short and stout. Here is my fang and here is my clout.

I'm a lit-tle mon-ster, cross-eyed too, and When I turn my eyes in, you turn to glue.
When I turn my eyes in, I'm scar-ing you.

When I keep my eyes straight the sky turns blue!

somehow equals the first Beach Ball. When this occurs, smoosh the two Beach Balls together with passion, with a sound—with an explosion or an implosion. Bring your smooshed Beach Balls to your heart and release them.

Have a good time with the song on page 185.

---

## Timetable for Strabismus

### Birth to One Year

Occasionally hold your hand over your baby's straight eye—only for as long as she will tolerate it. Use directional tromboning, Who's That in the Mirror?, songs, and finger plays.

### One to Five Years +

From the age of imitation (ten to twenty-four months) onward, patching should be a social affair. Other family members can use patches while games are played. As soon as the patch is bothersome, it comes off or sits on the top of the head. Using this approach, children have carried patches to their parents saying, "Let's sing 'Heave Ho!'" and "Aren't you going to use your patch?"

### Five Years +

Use Directional Tromboning, Photographing the Light, and the Windmill Swing.

---

# Heading for Fusion

All the directional games in this chapter are preparation for binocular vision, or fusion. You must decide when your child is ready to play the fusion games in the next chapter. You don't want to rush matters, but it may occur faster than you think. Follow your intuition. Most likely you and your child will be shifting back and forth between directional games, Patching, and fusion activities.

# 17

# Fusion

## What Is Fusion?

Fusion is binocular, or two-eyed, vision. It occurs when the messages from both eyes are used together by the visual brain. Only the images from the macula lutea are fused. Even though you don't notice, all contours and shapes peripheral to your small area of central fused vision are double. Hold the tip of your finger about fifteen centimeters (six inches) in front of your nose. Center your attention on your fingertip. Notice that all the other objects in the room, all the items you're not looking at, are double. They will be double unless you are using the message from only one of your eyes.

## The Physical Side of Fusion

The illustration at right shows how optic nerves connect eyeballs to the visual cortex in the back of the head.

Notice that the optic nerves meet at the optic chiasm. Here they shake hands and trade some nerve fibers, but only those from one side of their respective visual fields. Part of the visual field from the right eye leads to the left side of the visual cortex, and part of the visual field from the left eye leads to the right side of the visual cortex. The result? The left visual cortex gets handed the messages from the right side of the visual field from both your left and your right eye, and vice versa. Are you confused? It's an intriguing design. It works just fine until stress or trauma interferes.

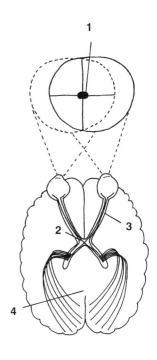

1 Macula lutea, the small area of fused and nuclear vision

2 Optic chiasm

3 Optic nerve

4 Primary visual cortex where fusion takes place

## Reasons for Not Fusing

Accident or disease can destroy fusion ability. If the eyes are physically healthy but there is a turned eye, the image from a turning eye may be put on hold by the brain. This was explained in the previous chapter on strabismus.

Since fusion is mainly directed from the brain, a restriction or illness that interferes with normal brain development could sabotage fusion. Another reason could be a large difference in the refractive error of each eye.

There is an emotional and mental side to fusion. The process of regaining fusion brings up powerful feelings. These feelings and their companion memories may be a primary cause of continued resistance to fusion.

## Why Is Fusion Important?

Unbalanced fusion leads to eyestrain and fatigue. Physical energy is used in trying to force a misaligned eye to stay in line with its partner. Even when the brain decides to suppress the image from one eye, it must burn energy to do so (page 168).

Balanced binocular vision brings with it distinct advantages. Full three-dimensional perception comes from blending together the macula lutea ("nuclear") images from each eye, producing rich color vision and full depth perception. If there are refractive error differences in the eyes, strong fusion helps to neutralize the discrepancy. Persons with -5 diopters in one eye and -1 diopter in the other may benefit tremendously from fusion games. With few exceptions, two eyes see better together than each eye separately.

Disturbed fusion and the three common refractive errors—myopia, hyperopia, and astigmatism—are all the result of an imbalance somewhere in the child's being. Occasionally take all children through the four levels of fusion as a helpful adjunct to their programs for refractive error, even when fusion is not the main problem.

## When to Do Fusion Games

Most of the fusion games in this chapter require special time with your child. I consider them suitable for ages five and up. At least once a week you could say, "Let's meet Thursday evening to play fusion games at the kitchen table." If you can get in a second session on Sunday morning, that will be even better.

Once your child gets to the stage where he is familiar with fusion games, encourage him to teach them to other children. Young people are excellent teachers. Knowledge passed on solidifies in the giver.

Before you do fusion games together, warm up with Cross-Crawl dancing and Palming. Use Emotional Healing for fusion as needed. Adults have burst into tears on seeing with fusion for the first time in a vision class. Other students became cranky when they didn't get the Gate described below. Expect sparks and carry tissues.

When doing fusion games it is important to return continually to relaxation, Yawning, and Cross-Crawl. Use lots of praise and recognition of baby steps in healing fusion. If your child sees the Gate for half a second, pause for jubilation. That may even be enough success for one session.

Do not allow your disapproval of turned eyes to flavor the game. Keep yourself free of fairy-tale prejudices the best you can.

After all that—let's get to some action!

## Fusion Level One: The Gate

Place your finger about fifteen centimeters (six inches) directly in front of your nose. Edge something in the distance beyond your finger with your Magic Nose Pencil.

You may notice that your finger appears doubled and blurred. We call this phenomenon "the Gate." It comes when you have fusion, when you are using the images from both eyes.

If you do not have the Gate, you might be looking directly at your finger. Please send your attention into the distance. If your gate still doesn't appear, your visual brain may have turned off the image from one of your eyes.

Sometimes it takes a while for the second image to click in, so be patient with this if it doesn't occur right away.

If the second finger doesn't appear at all, see what happens with the

This FFF has a fish on one side and a fishbowl on the other.

Fantastic Fusion Fixer (FFF): Cut a piece of stiff cardboard about ten centimeters (four inches) wide and fifteen centimeters (six inches) long. The card should have complementary colors on the front and back sides for high contrast: bright red on one side, with the other side green; one side blue and the other orange; or yellow and purple. Pasting together two pieces of different-colored construction paper will do. You could also color or paint some white paper.

Glue a picture of a brilliant flower or animal to one side of the card. Make sure the image contrasts highly with the background color on that side of the card. Put a bee on the other side.

Hold the card perpendicular to your nose (see illustration), snug enough to your face so that your right eye sees only the right side of the card and your left eye sees only the left side of the card.

Will is looking at a flower in the distance through his FFF.

While holding the FFF card in front of your nose, cover your right eye with a hand or another card. Notice, absorb, and memorize the side of the card you see with your left eye. Alternately: Cover your left eye with your hand or another card. Notice, absorb, and memorize the side of the card you see with the open eye.

Close both eyes. With your eyes closed, remember and visualize the left eye's side of the card to the right of your nose. Visualize the right eye's side of the card to the left of your nose. Now *imagine the two sides of the card at the same time.* I agree it's tricky. The cards switch sides because your optic nerves trade fibers, as mentioned above.

Open both eyes. Say, "Hurrah!" if both sides of the card, the bee and the flower, appear at the same time, even for a split second. Repeat this activity at other times until you have a solid, lasting experience of binocular vision.

## Straight Eyes but No Fusion?

It is possible to have both eyes straight, with no large difference in the refractive error of the two eyes, but still not have fusion. The message from one eye is being used; the other message is playing second fiddle. In this case Patching is helpful to encourage the eye that is not being fully utilized to catch up.

## Deciding Which Eye to Patch

When there is a turning eye, it is easy to determine which eye to patch. The patch goes on the straight eye. In the case where it is not so obvious, use the Fantastic Fusion Fixer to discover which eye is not being used. Switch the card around several times, letting each eye have a chance to view the flower. If the flower consistently *disappears when it's on the right side* of your nose, then your brain may be turning off the messages from your right eye. Therefore you would *patch your left eye*.

If the flower consistently *disappears on the left side* of your nose, then your brain may be turning off the messages from your left eye. Therefore you would *patch your right eye*.

Cover up the "good eye" and play some movement vision games for a while. If you do put on an eye patch, fusion games won't work, because you will only get fusion if you have two uncovered functioning eyes. After Patching for a while, return to fusion games and see what happens.

##  Fusion Level Two: The Bug and Bead Game

Take a piece of string about two meters (six feet) long. One person holds each end of the string, or tie one end to a convenient structure. You should end up sitting about one meter (three feet) away from where the string is fastened to the other person, a chair, or a railing. Wind your end of the string around your forefinger and hold it fifteen centimeters (six inches) in front of your chin. Don't hold the string too tightly to your chin. You want to be able to move your head around easily.

Place a brightly colored bead on your string. If two people are holding the string, each will have her own bead. If you can't find a bead in your house, use a paper clip, a small hair band, a piece of thick yarn, or a diamond ring. Slide the bead outward until it is sitting twenty-five centimeters (ten inches) from your hand.

Now that you are all set with your string and bead, close your eyes and pretend you have a pet bug flying around in the room. It could be a bee, a butterfly, a pterodactyl, a spaceship, or whatever you like. Your bug or UFO loves aerial acrobatics. It performs loop-the-loops and triple somersaults with the greatest of ease. You follow your bug with your nose of course. (This can be done first with a real object, a toy for example, until you have the idea, then use your imagination.)

Fuchsia's bug landed on her bead. So did both her eyes.

After your bug has finished showing off, it will come in for a landing exactly on your bead.

Blink your eyes open and circle the bug on your bead with your nose. What do you notice? Do you have one string or two? Has the string you are holding with one hand magically made itself into two strings? If it has, then you are experiencing fusion—which can now be refined with the next question.

Are the two strings meeting and making an X somewhere near your bead with the bug on it?

*Case 1.* If your X crosses within two and a half centimeters (one inch) in front of your bead, your mind and your eye muscles are working together.

Congratulations. Grasp the bead with your free hand and give your bug a ride near and far on the string. Breathe and yawn. This near-far movement with the bead combines both fusion and accommodation. Excellent for reading stamina and a career in computers. Repeat this game only occasionally.

*Case 2.* If your X is crossing more than five centimeters (two inches) *in front of* your bug, put your string down and Trombone out and to the side, favoring the phoria, for three minutes. Time's up? Stop Tromboning, pick up your string, and see if your X is now crossing closer to your bead. Yes? Congratulations. If you don't know already what Tromboning is from chapter 16, here it is.

A Tromboning paddle

## Tromboning Outward for Esophoria

Make yourself a paddle of stiff cardboard. Put some brightly colored stickers or cutouts on the paddle to attract the eye. Because eyes are always attracted to motion and color, we move the paddle like the slide on a trombone to coax a turned or wandering eye in the direction we want it to go. With Tromboning, overtight muscles relax. (See instructions on page 176.)

For eyes that tend to pull too far inward, the paddle is used to escort the eye in an outward direction. Covering the opposite eye with the palm of the hand, trombone the paddle from your nose outward, away from the center/midline of your body. Humming and crooning will help to stimulate the visual system while easing the eye outward. Change eyes and do the same movement. Do each eye for about three minutes. (See illustration on page 177, figures C and D.)

## The Widening River

The Widening River visualization is helpful for eyes that are overconverging. These eyes are called esophoric. Esophoria does not have to be so severe as to be labeled strabismus. It is, however, a subtle tendency that can result in brain and eye fatigue.

Put the string and bead away for a while. Palm your eyes and tell a story where you imagine you are standing at the source of a river. The river widens as it flows away in front of you. Trace the side of the river extending out to the right and then the side extending to the left. Fill out your visualization of the river with fish, turtles, and charming mermaids. Two mermaids swim away from you. They get farther away from one another as they swim into the distance. They find their sitting rocks on the horizon and wave at you. After Palming go back to the Bug and Bead.

*Case 3.* If your X crosses beyond your bead or you have two parallel lines, then it's time to stop and do some Tromboning inward for three minutes. Then return to the bead and string to see if your X has moved closer to your bead.

## Tromboning Inward for Exophoria

For eyes that tend to drift outward, cover one eye and hold the paddle in front of you. Trombone the paddle in and out, crossing the midline of your body, noticing the pictures getting larger and smaller. Hum with the in-and-out rhythm of your paddle. Humming sounds vibrate skull bones and activate your right brain. The paddle attracts and coaxes the eye inward. Do the same action with your other eye.

Do Tromboning for about three minutes. (See illustrations on page 177, figures A and B.)

## The Precious Shell

Visualizing the Precious Shell will help loosen eye muscles and tell your brain it's okay to point both your eyes toward the bead at the same time. Put the string and bead aside for a moment. Palm your eyes and imagine you are at the seashore. You stand at the edge of the water looking out toward the ocean. In the distance on your right is a mermaid sitting on a rock. Her twin sister is sitting on a rock in the distance to your left. When you whistle, they both jump into the water and swim toward you as fast as they can. They are converging on

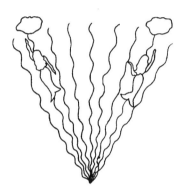

The mermaids swim away from you if your eye goes inward.

The mermaids swim toward you if your eye goes outward.

you. Smiling, their hair dripping seaweed, they each hand you half a seashell. You must put the two halves of the seashell together right in front of your eyes.

Once your seashell is together, put it in your pocket. Bring your palms away from your face, blink your eyes open, and return to your string. Is your X now closer to your bead? Congratulations.

If at any time you find you have stiffened up your shoulders, or if you're turning blue from holding your breath, please take a break. Yawn like a lion. Do Cross-Crawl dancing before returning to the Bug and Bead.

*Note to adults:* When playing the Bug and Bead game with a younger child, please do not ask him if he has an X. Phrase the question differently. Ask him what he sees as he holds the string and circles the bug. Once you have a response, you can go from there: "How many strings do you have?" and "Show me with your free hand where the strings go." If he sees two strings (which may or may not cross), you can ask, "Do the two strings meet anywhere?" and "Where do they cross?"

## Fusion Level Three: Fish in a Bowl

More fusion fun can be had by children who are already seeing the Gate at least part of the time if they use fusion cards they have made themselves. Using these cards will help their visual brain get more into the fusion habit.

On a plain piece of paper or card just the right size to hold in your hand, draw a fishbowl on the left side and a fish on the right side. Draw the pictures four centimeters (about one and a half inches) apart because that is the easiest distance for the visual system to overlap two images when the card is held twenty-five centimeters (ten inches) in front of your nose.

At first you may get four images, two fish and two fishbowls. Realize that it may take a few moments for the fish to overlap with the fishbowl. Breathe,

Fusion cards by
NVI teacher
Shirley Beasley

4 cm

smile, and move the card slowly near and far until you hear a splash.

The possibilities for fusion-card creations are infinite. Make a deck of cards with sport, cooking, or musical themes. Let yourselves brainstorm ideas. In brainstorming, every idea is accepted, so stir up as many ideas as possible—the wilder the better.

## Fusion Level Four: Magic Eyes

When children have a lot of reading and desk work to do or are sitting at computers, their visual system needs *fusion reserve*. This means their brain-and-eye-muscle coordination has such a strong foundation that even hours of reading (with the Great White Glow) will not make their eyes tired or strained.

The popular "Magic Eye" books and posters are based on this principle.

From *The Magic Eye*, N. E. Thing Enterprises

Two kinds of haloes

A child who does not have solid fusion abilities will be left out in the cold when others are exclaiming over the 3-D images that are emerging from the garbled computer-generated graphics.

But once he has developed the Gate and progressed through fusion levels two and three, he should (with relaxation and gentle scanning with his Magic Nose Feather) be able to satisfy his heart.

### Angel Haloes

Once your child has achieved fusion level one—the Gate—you can make him an Angel Halo. There are several ways to make a Halo. You could use pipe cleaners or soft clothesline wire. But please do not put the metal circle all the way around the head, as you would be closing off the governing meridian, causing mental scramble and discomfort. We use a rubber band to close the V front of a metal Halo that encircles the head.

An alternative is to make a hole in the bill of a baseball cap and push a straight stick through the hole. Children can wear the Halo when reading or doing any other activity. It is especially good for hyperopic children to build fusional reserve.

The vertical part of the Halo should sit at a distance from the child's eyes where the two sides of the Gate fall into the margin of the page. Use the Halo while doing the Bird Swing to multiply saccadic movement.

Fuchsia is using a wire Halo under her baseball cap.

## Alternating Vision

Alternating strabismus, or squint, occurs when the child looks at you with the right eye, sending the left eye off to the woods, then looks at you with the left eye, sending the right eye off for a swim. Alternating vision is trainable. With loving persistence you have a good chance of inviting errant eyes back to the same party. Patching will not help in this case. But fusion games with lots of body feeling, excitement, and enthusiasm will call in the two eyes to land on your face at the same time.

The following fusion games are based on the irresistible power of imagination and body awareness, the kind we get from swinging on a swing or dancing. Touching hands and eyes will feed back into the visual brain what it is like to use the messages from both eyes simultaneously.

## ◉ The Butterfly Mask

*Materials needed.* Paper, crayons, Scotch tape, rubber bands or string to fasten the mask on the child's head.

The illustration shown is an example. Your child could make his own mask. Perhaps he prefers the face of a lion or a *Tyrannosaurus rex*.

Cut two eye holes for the mask, making sure they are right in front of the child's eyes. While holding his right hand in yours, ask him to find you with his right eye. Holding his left hand in yours, ask him to find you with his left eye. Do this several times until you are fairly sure he is aware of which eye he is using. Bring both his hands together saying, "Find me with both eyes at once." Give a jubilant *ahhh*, whether he succeeds or not.

How many times you might be able to repeat this game I don't know. I do know that any kind of change takes love and patience. Be assured that your child's brain will be mulling over the possibilities. Do this game for three minutes each time—longer if he wants to.

## 👁 Candles in the Dark

*Materials needed.* Two candles, a colored sticker to put on your nose, a darkened room. (*Note:* Two penlights would work equally well.)

1. In your darkened room hold two lit candles about fifteen centimeters (six inches) in front of your child and about five centimeters (two inches) apart. Put a sticker or a colored mark on the end of your nose. Tell the child, "This is what you will see when you are fusing."

   Now hold one candle in front of him and say, "This one light will magically turn into two candles like this." Again hold up the two candles about five centimeters (two inches) apart. All the time, he is circling the sticker on your nose, not looking at the candle or penlight.

2. Hold one candle about fifteen centimeters (six inches) in front of his nose. Have your child close his eyes and imagine the two flames of the candles while circling the sticker on your nose in his mind.

3. While still imagining the two flames, the child opens his eyes.

4. If he sees two flames with his eyes open even for an instant, everybody celebrate. Celebrate even if he doesn't see two flames or lights. Perhaps next time.

## ◉ Feeling Fusion

By using whole-body movement together with imagination activities, we can help encourage the brain to fuse the images from the two eyes. First, cut two strips of paper about five centimeters (two inches) wide. Have your child draw and color an eye on each piece of paper. Wrap the paper eyes around his hand and fasten them with adhesive tape. Attune the left hand to the left eye by repeating phrases such as: "This is your left hand. With your left hand you can see by touching things." Touch a flower or a rock or a piece of toast or a cool breeze. Then touch the left hand to the left eye and explore eyelid, eyelashes, and eyebrow with the fingers of the left hand.

Repeat this action with the right hand and eye: "This is your right hand. With your right hand you can see by touching things. Touch a piece of wood, my nose, the water in this glass."

Second, discover what is the child's favorite kind of thing for the day—cars, rabbits, airplanes, fairies? Now make a cardboard box into a home or haven for the child's favorite things, by cutting a suitably shaped opening at the front, and drawing and coloring on the remaining area. For example, make a garage for the cars with a large doorway, windows, lanterns, and grass and flowers on the front. The rabbits might live in a rabbit hole, the fairies might live in a flower, the airplanes might have a hangar or a Fusion Bay! The opening should be large enough for the child to put both hands in.

Now draw images of the chosen objects on strips which you will wrap around the child's hands or wrists and tape or tie on. Make one object for each hand. Have the child play with each object separately first: "This car is your left eye car, it drives around like this, *vroom vroom*." Then, "This car is your right eye car, it drives around like this, *vroom, vroom*." Next the hands come and play together, then go together into the hole in the box. "Now your two eye cars drive together, and go together into their garage like this! Yay!" Make a happy fuss about the hands doing their thing together.

You can create rhymes as you do the actions:

| | | |
|---|---|---|
| My right eye is a rabbit, | or | My right eye is an airplane, |
| My left eye is a hare. | | My left eye is one too. |
| When they see their hole— | | When they see Fusion Bay— |
| They both jump right in there | | They fly into the blue! |

Use the hands again to get the feeling of fusion deep, deep into the body and mind. In your left hand is a lake. Close your eyes and imagine the lake. In your right hand is a moon. The moon and the lake splash together. In your left hand is a red banana pie. In your right hand is a blue banana pie. Squish the two pies together. What do you get?

At another time you can imagine your two hands are lanterns glowing fiercely outdoors on a dark windy night. Take a big breath and bring the two glowing lamps together. What do you get?

If your child is old enough, you could experiment with bringing together the flames of two candles. First for real, then in the imagination. Always do the motions with hands and arms even when imagining. The kinesthetic movement of the body feeds the feeling of fusion into the brain.

After tuning up body and brain for fusion, take the child with alternating vision back to level one—the Gate. See what happens.

If you and your child dream up new ideas and games for finding fusion, please send them to the Center. Your ideas will be shared with other families.

## ◉ Emotional Healing for Fusion

The essence of fusion is joining together and cooperation. The right eye and right side of the body directed through the left brain represent the male aspect and father. Mother and the feminine are represented by the left eye and left side of the body and the right brain. Male and female union within one-self is as vulnerable to disruption as getting married in America. One out of three unions end in divorce. Cameron Dawson finds that 30 percent of his patients have fusion problems ranging from hardly noticeable to grossly strabismic.

Statements to play with:

| | |
|---|---|
| I see with one eye. | I see with both eyes. |
| I am cockeyed. | My eyes are balanced. |

There is a silent internal argument going on. When this conflict is made audible it sounds something like this:

| | |
|---|---|
| I want to be separate. | I want to join together. |
| I must be single. | I am everything. |
| I will be destroyed by others. | Others uplift me. |
| I must look out for myself. | I am safe. |

Use Melting Beach Balls to clarify and dissolve blocked feelings. Not every child will have the same thought patterns. Start out simply by placing the fact in your left hand: "I see with one eye." Make it into an energy ball with color, size, and weight. Repeat the words out loud with enthusiasm, making your Beach Ball grow in size and effect until the rocks and oceans notice it. Now ask the question: "Can you love yourself even when you see with one eye?" If the answer is yes, then ask for the opposite of seeing with one eye. Put that response in a huge Beach Ball in your right hand: "I see with both eyes together at the same time." Build up this statement with color and impact. When your two balls balance each other and you are satisfied with your expressions, implode your two balls together right in front of you. Bring your hands to your heart and go on with your life.

---

## Timetable for Fusion

### Birth to Eight Months

During this homolateral phase it's too early for fusion games. Do swinging and directional games if your baby has a turned eye.

### Eight Months to One Year

This is the building and solidifying phase for fusion. In general, sit back and watch the baby crawl in his own time. If your child needs help, you can do manual Cross-Crawling. You grasp his right hand and bring it to his left foot and vice versa. Do this not more than ten times in a session.

### Two to Four Years

Continue with directional Tromboning and swings (if needed) from chapter 16.

### Four to Six Years

Experiment with the Gate, using yardsticks, colored pens, and home-made fusion cards.

### Six to Ten Years +

Start with the Gate, then go on to fusion level two, the Bug and Bead game. Take children slowly and patiently through fusion levels one to four. Return frequently to easy fusion games where kids can be successful. Edge yourselves slowly and delicately toward more advanced levels.

Part 4

# Home and School Environments

# 18

# Sugar and Sore Eyes

## Bodies Are Made of Food

Just as a factory needs raw materials to produce a go-cart or a computer, children need raw materials of a particular kind to produce healthy body parts. Vitamins, minerals, and proteins are the necessary ingredients. Every newborn is gifted with an immense ability to recover. Every child comes in with reservoirs of enzymes and minerals. The diet of the mother while pregnant has an effect; and what goes into the child's body in the next years will determine her moods and affect her physical health. If she lives on empty calories, her reservoirs will be depleted rather than replenished.

It looks as if children can eat anything. They have strong digestions, pink cheeks, and bounding energy. Sometimes it takes twelve years of junk food to produce a teenager with poor eyesight, sugar addiction (which has been linked to teenage alcoholism, a major problem in the United States), depression, and problems in school.

The person buying the groceries determines the diet patterns of the rest of the family. Starting children out with foods that contain the building blocks for the body is a challenge. Do what you can before and during the high chair phase. You will have to educate relatives and friends who come offering sweets. This requires daily practice. It will take shopping-bag awareness. It could mean changing what you eat.

A thorough discussion of foods and their relationship to the eye, brain, and mind complex would require another book. I had to decide on a key element: white sugar. Why do I pick on white sugar?

Sugar is the ultimate challenge. Having raised three children in a sugar culture, I know the pitfalls and opposing forces. If you can divert (or even blow up) the sugar train, promoting any other healthy dietary habits will be easy. If you as a parent or caregiver to children can produce a child who will buy an apple rather than a candy bar, I salute you. At fifteen she may be making salads and steaming vegetables without being asked. Another reason I have chosen white sugar is that white sugar has been linked to developing myopia.

## Sugar Blues

The World Health Organization has listed processed sugar as one of the five substances to which citizens of industrial nations are addicted. Dare I call processed sugar a drug? My dictionary says a drug is a chemical substance taken for the pleasant effect it produces. I learned, when first giving weekend vision-improvement seminars, to ask the organizers to whisk away the coffee and sugar packets.

"Also get rid of these cookies and sweet biscuits!" I didn't quite bellow. All my myopic students were nodding off at three o'clock in the afternoon. When I spoke of sugar highs and sugar lows, a sixteen-year-old protested, "I thought sugar gives you energy." Yes, for a short period, then it opens a trapdoor under your feet. Simple sugar overstimulates the pancreas. Complex sugars, as found in fruits and vegetables, stay with you longer. The pancreas is related to feelings of apathy: "I just can't move." On the second day of the seminar apples and oranges were served.

Excessive sugar in the body is eliminated partially through the eyes. "Sleep" (the crystalline crust found in your eyes in the morning) is often caused by the sweets you ate yesterday.

This drug is not an outlaw. It's everywhere. In relation to vision problems it is our first and main wrestling partner.

Your child's visual field is plastered with the shape, color, and taste of soft drinks and candy. Chocolate, cheap and exclusive, is the taste that consoles, congratulates, and celebrates. Let's take a look at chocolate candy bars in relationship to the visual blur called myopia.

All chocolate contains white sugar and oxalic acid. White sugar in the body sneaks into its mineral storehouse and steals away chromium. What's chromium? It's a trace mineral. Lack of chromium is a factor in the development of myopia.

Oxalic acid slows down the rate at which calcium is absorbed in the body. Calcium is essential for strong teeth and bones. It's the reason we are told to drink our milk. Yet the calcium in milk is insoluble in the human body. Cow's milk products have had excellent press and advertising. More people are finding out that they are not fit for human consumption. The chocolate milk we were given in our school lunches contained the worst of both worlds. One sign of lack of calcium is increased myopia.

It is an illusion to increase the intake of calcium-bearing foods such as milk and cheese in the hope that your body will take calcium out of these foods and put it in the right places. Calcium works in partnership with magnesium. Some doctors believe that high calcium intake of the wrong kind causes premature aging, premenstrual tension, and osteoporosis. Rather than forcing ice cream, cheese, and milk down children, it is advised to increase magnesium. One of the best ways to do this is to cook peasant food for your family. This means foods like whole-grain millet, barley, and rye. Millet contains eight parts magnesium to one part calcium. Use these grains cooked as breakfast cereals. After soaking grains overnight, use them sprouted and mixed with veggies as cold salads.

# Sugar Hit Parade

The child's world is sprinkled with white sugar: cakes, cookies, and candy bars. "Empty calories," they are called, for they have no bodybuilding value. In my dream I entered our local general store. Glitter and sparkle, purple, green, gold, dazzled my eyes from the floor to eight feet. Inside the glitzy flat or lumpy parcels were nuggets of sweet brownness. Three girls, just losing their baby teeth, stood at the counter with sweaty pocket coins in one hand, their selections in the other. Doing research for this book, I asked them why they were spending their pocket money on candy. A blue-eyed blondy replied, "It's got tattoos in it." The second grinned. "I can win a prize." The third little girl glared at me. "I like the taste."

You must cope with advertisements on TV, birthday parties, school parties, and festivals. Soft drinks can contain up to 60 percent white sugar. What can you do? Gain some understanding of the chemical and emotional significance of sugar consumption. Then find and use at home and school as many substitution ideas as possible.

Emotionally, sugar is the taste of the past. It soothes and pacifies like suckling at the breast. Chocolate stimulates endorphins, which are chemical relaxants and pleasure hormones in the brain. Sugar is a drug that reminds people of past comforts. It is eaten by people yearning for love. Chocolate contains caffeine, a stimulant and toxin. That's a double whammy surrogate adventure story that ends in a crumbling crystal palace. It's a transitory addictive illusion that weakens bodies and minds. One therapy for addictions is to overdo it. Try living only on chocolate for a couple of weeks, observing your behavior and thoughts. Or consider taking in minerals.

## Why People Want Sugar

People who crave sugar are *lacking in minerals*. Refined and processed foods, such as cakes, candies, cookies, cereals, white rice, and white bread, have been stripped of vitamins and minerals. Foods grown on soil replenished only with phosphate and nitrogenous fertilizers are lacking in trace minerals.

It's a vicious circle. The child is missing minerals and experiences this lack as a longing for sugar. Sugar enters the bloodstream, giving a rise in energy. Children call this a sugar hit. Blood sugar levels rise rapidly, triggering an alarm that races through the body crying out "Too much sugar here. Get rid of it." The body obeys and blood sugar drops suddenly. Your marvelous, vital angel transforms into a tired rag doll or an irritable brat.

The culprit being discussed here is refined white sugar. More complex sugars such as those in fruit and fruit juices do not cause the same highs and lows in blood sugar levels that white sugar does. "Why does Steve have constant headaches?" his mother asked me after a vision class. I turned around and asked ten-year-old Steve, "How much soda pop are you drinking?" "Two bottles of Pepsi a day," he said. When fruit juice was substituted for the sugared carbonated water, Steve's headaches stopped. Vegetables and grains contain complex carbohydrates (sugar and starch molecules) that take even longer to break down in the body. These are the foods that "stay with" you.

# What You Can Do

Complaining doesn't work. "You're eating too much candy" can bring out a rebel response.

What works is to eat right yourself—at least during the age of imitation, which is birth to age five. During this time eating habits are established. Baby Aerro was fed mainly vegetables, whole-cooked grains, and fruit. On his first birthday the celebrating adults decided to buy a chocolate cake, something Aerro had never seen. A piece was put in his mouth. Everyone laughed at the wry expression on his face. Aerro spurned more cake and crawled over to my plate to gobble up green peas.

Get minerals into your body. Vegetables and whole grains contain minerals. If you live in a region where you suspect the vegetables are grown on depleted soil, then consider buying a mineral supplement. Ask at your health food store or drugstore for a mineral supplement that would be suitable for both you and your child.

Fill your shopping bag with fresh fruit and vegetables rather than squishy things in shiny, colored wrappers. Yes, our eyes are attracted to glitz, but also to bright oranges and slippery bananas.

Buy unsweetened fruit juices and dilute to a proportion of two parts juice to one part water. Freeze this into ice cubes in summer.

Look for recipe books on healthy food for children.

People with hypoglycemia (low blood sugar) are told to eat protein rather than simple sugars. There is lots of protein in nuts and seeds. To restore enzyme activity, soak sunflower seeds, almonds, hazelnuts, or peanuts in water overnight or for six hours. Pour the water off and rinse in a sieve. Keep them in the refrigerator if they are not eaten up the first day. They are crunchy, fulfilling, and visually interesting. They start to grow.

For snacks, carry apples, oranges, carrots, celery, rice crackers, nuts, dates, and raisins.

As sweeteners use "real" sugars such as honey (remembering that some people cannot use honey because it is too concentrated), maple syrup, dates, and rice and apple syrup.

See if you can get school chocolate sales turned into flower sales. Imagine my delight: flower bulb companies are now prepared to help schools raise funds by turning children into daffodil sellers instead of candy vendors. There are now candy-free checkout lines in some American supermarkets.

## I'D LIKE TO BE

*Words and Music by Donald Woodward*

Add your own rhymes about fruit and vegetables you like!

## A Good Start

Here is Aerro's eating story from his mother:

I knew that I wanted Aerro to start out with a good strong nutritional base. I knew for this to happen I wanted him to get a taste for vegetables rather than sweets. I heard that if babies are introduced to sweet foods first, they refuse vegetables. I think his first food other than breast milk was at four or five months. He was given diluted fresh vegetable juice in a bottle (carrot and celery). He loved it. Then I gave him mixtures of veggie and apple juice. His first solid food was steamed veggies mushed up. Then mashed banana.

As his teeth started to come in he got more solid foods, but always cooked grains (he loves rice) or mashed veggies or mashed fresh fruit. When he started teething more, he was made very happy by crackers to chew on. I gave him plain crackers without sugar and with little salt, such as rice cakes, rice crackers, or Ryvita. I have found to this day that he is always happy to eat simple foods. Toast with no butter, plain crackers, and veggies with no salt (although he likes stir-fry with soy sauce or noodle-and-veggie soup with flavor). He has been exposed to cheese-flavored chips, the joy of cookies, and other goodies. He loves these too, and his eyes light up when he sees a junk food packet. But he will still, at two years old, happily eat plain steamed vegetables and rice and loves fresh fruit.

He was never given cow's milk at home. But he loves goat's yogurt and sometimes goat cheese. The occasional times he has gotten a bit of cow's milk or cheese, I've immediately seen him with a runny nose for a day or two. I have noticed one other thing. Where normally he wouldn't eat alfalfa sprouts, one time we were out and had only french fries for lunch. I went and bought a container of alfalfa sprouts to eat with it, as I feel sick eating only greasy food. Well, Aerro asked for and ate up a good amount of those sprouts. I know he normally wouldn't, but I felt that he knew on some level that he wanted that green to help his tummy with the grease.

I have noticed a big difference from other kids who were brought up on manufactured baby foods, which are full of sugar and salt. These mothers with one-year-olds with spotty faces remark on how healthy Aerro looks and how healthy his skin looks. These children also seem to be very picky about what they eat. They only want food with tons of flavor, salty or sweet. Many parents are amazed when they see Aerro eating exactly what I eat instead of special food prepared for a picky child. I know he will be exposed to and probably eat lots of unhealthy food in his life. But I am very happy to know that he will happily and of his own choice eat healthy food as well.

## Emotional Healing for Sugar Freaks

Use the Melting Beach Balls technique to find a way out of the sugar addiction and apathy maze.

Some familiar thought and word patterns:

| | |
|---|---|
| I can't see anyway. | I'm able to see. |
| I'm too tired. | I'm full of energy. |
| I don't matter. | I'm important. |
| I learned it but I can't use it. | I use everything. |
| I'd rather just sit here. | I love to move. |

Put the words "I can't see" in your right-hand Beach Ball. We'd better get a bicycle pump for this one. Getting enthusiastic about apathy is hard. You feel like you're encased in a heavy lead diving suit. Let's go diving then. The Beach Ball that says "I can't see" is getting bigger and heavier and heavier. It's carrying you down and down into the dark mud. Here we are. How does it feel? Is it okay to be sunk in apathy, *in the can'ts:* "I can't do, can't see, can't breathe, can't move"? Can you give yourself a teeny ray of light down here? Think about it. Imagine it. Yes?

Let's ask ourselves, "What is the opposite of 'I can't see'? 'You're able to see'?" Is that okay too? That Beach Ball in your left hand is getting bigger. You're blowing it up with the bicycle pump? With your lungs? It's going to be tricky bringing that heavy lead ball and the airy light ball together. You'll find a way? Wonder-full! Now sing the song on page 209 with great enthusiasm.

# 19

# Your Child's Room

Room designs and furnishings can remind, inspire, and entice children to do vision games when they are alone. Place your homemade vision charts in strategic places; put nature posters and infinity signs over desks where schoolwork is done.

Right

Wrong

## Lighting, Computers, Homework

Fluorescent lighting—even when it is the new "broad spectrum" lighting—still flickers at a frequency that is disturbing to the human organism. It has been shown to promote myopia. For these reasons I recommend incandescent or halogen lightbulbs.

The light should fall directly downward onto your child's work or come from the side. The computer screen should be placed against a wall. If there is a light source from a lamp or window behind the screen, eyestrain results. Your child's eyes are attracted to the light source even when his mind is trying to stay on the screen.

Keeping your Magic Paintbrush moving across the computer screen will help prevent the development of "computer eyes." Paint the background color of the screen with the Paintbrush. A wonderful habit for computer users to get into is Palming at the workstation.

Prop your elbows on the desk and Palm for several seconds while the hard drive is making its maneuvers. Moving your attention near and far flexes the muscles of accommodation. The NVI poster with eagle and crocodile (see page 240) provides a long road for Near-Far Swings at your desk. This poster features six vision games, including Painting White and Counting Cactus.

Ergonomics, the study of the relationship between workers and their environment, dictates that when using a computer, both feet should be on the floor and the spine erect. Hands and forearms on keyboards need to make a 90-degree angle with upper arms and shoulders. The Occupational Health and Safety Unit in Australia recommends a break from computer work every fifteen minutes. If your child spends hours glued to a video or computer screen, work out a plan with him to do any of the vision games from this book at fifteen- to thirty-minute intervals.

# Design a Vision Nest for Eaglets

The following room designs were devised during a Vision Improvement Playcamp held for children and their parents at the community house of Crystal Waters Permaculture Village. Optometric reports and life histories for the children were sent to us before the Playcamp started.

During the five days of the camp, we played vision games together, tailoring them to different ages and eyesight problems. Emotional Healing sessions were first held with parents, who were overcontrolling their children's play. After releasing the pressure that their kids must exactly obey and instantly see better, we all relaxed.

The last day of the camp the children and teachers drew up room plans. We decided where the theme eye charts would go on the wall, where the trampoline would be put, and what rug they could lie on for Palming.

The following examples are all by hyperopic children. A room designed for a myopic child would be similar except that a young myope needs vistas. A Bug and Bead game attached to a windowsill would allow him to take fusion and Near-Far Swings outward into the landscape. Posters of oceans, skylines, and mountain ranges could decorate his walls, providing settings for long-range visual journeys.

## Jack's Room (Age Eight)

The design team asked a number of questions, which were repeated for each child. Jack's history was considered first.

Jack's mother believed his brain damage had been caused by a triple antigen vaccination at six months. His left brain was affected, resulting in partial lameness on the right side of his body. Jack had a lazy left eye and had gone through two sets of prescription glasses for hyperopia to use at school. He refused to do eye exercises. "He was sick of all the doctors," his mother reported. In November of 1993 an optometrist had measured his vision at

+2.25 with -0.50 x 180-degree axis. A pediatric ophthalmologist in October 1993 had measured Jack's vision at +6.75 with -2.00 x 10 degrees and +7.25 with -1.5 at 175-degree axis. Just before coming to the Vision Playcamp, Jack had expressed, in the words of his mother, "dissatisfaction with his physical drawbacks."

Q. Teachers, what are the important games for Jack to play?

A. He needs lots of movement for hyperopia and Patching to bring his left eye outward. Use the Bug and Bead game to solidify the fusion he achieved during Playcamp fusion games, plus lots of Cross-Crawling activities for his brain.

Q. Jack, what are your favorite vision games?

A. Ball games and crawling games.

Q. What sort of ball games?

A. Soccer and football.

At home Jack shared a room with his two younger sisters while his parents were building an extension. The room we drew with Jack on a huge piece of paper looks like this.

Jack's room

## Daniel's Room (Age Six)

The history report from Daniel's mother told us that he had a brain seizure in August of 1989 and was revived by ambulance staff. He had glasses for hyperopia since his vision problem was picked up by the preschool nurse. His lenses had been strengthened three times. He was reversing some letters and his mom said his handwriting was terrible. An eye surgeon had measured Daniel's vision at +6.00 and +7.00. In February 1994 a behavioral optometrist measured his eyes at +5.50 and +5.50. She sent me a thorough, typed visual assessment for the Playcamp. She found Daniel had no depth perception up close, and that with his glasses on his convergence was good.

Q.   Teachers, what are the important vision games for Daniel to play?
A.   As a hyperope Daniel needs his left brain switched on and movement to break the stare, especially up close. He loves the Ball on the String and the Bug and Bead games. He uses a Halo when he does his Bird Swing to increase saccadic movement.
Q.   Daniel, what do you like most in your life?
A.   Viruses.

Daniel had watched a TV program on viruses. He loves viruses. Therefore you have the privilege of seeing Daniel's renderings of viruses in this book.

Six weeks after the Playcamp: "Daniel is no longer dependent on glasses. When his T-Glasses broke he put on his old prescription. They gave him headaches and sore eyes. He is doing most of the activities on most days and lots of Cross-Crawling. His handwriting has improved after working with an Edu-K counselor." His mother, Mandy, introduced the Rainbow Ribbon Wand to the first grade class at their public school, with the principal's approval. The principal had to try it out himself first. Mandy is pleased with Daniel's progress. Daniel is happy.

I wish to share the most up-to-date report from Mandy. "Whom can I tell? I am so excited and fired up. We've really achieved something." I ask, "Please tell me slowly Mandy, what happened?" "Because you had called and asked how Daniel was doing, I took him back to the optometrist sooner than I had planned. She tested him and smiled. "Very nice changes in both eyes," she said. He was reading two lines better on the visual acuity test. He was passing the first test in depth perception. And his vision measured at +3.25 in both eyes. That's less than his original preschool prescription of +4.00 and +3.75."

"Which activities have you been doing?" I asked.

"He's using the Swinging Ball right now. He uses his pin-holes on the computer. We do lots of Cross-Crawling. He's almost seven and he will do these things without being nagged. His Rainbow Ribbon Wand is around here somewhere."

I asked to speak with Daniel to get the story from the lion's mouth. "I've been doing that Ball Swing for a long time. Mummy does a sneaky Cross-Crawl with one finger and one toe." When I asked Daniel how his viruses were doing, he said, "I hate nightmares." I suggested that when he sees a scary image in his dream that he assert, "This is my dream, what are you doing here?"

Daniel's room

## Leanne's Room (Age Nine)

Leanne joined our ChildVision Playcamp accompanied by her mother, Yvonne. She had been prescribed glasses six weeks previously by a behavioral optometrist. There was a delay in obtaining her diagnosis on paper. Her mother had not understood the jargon used by the optometrist. In the meantime, Yvonne decided to experience NVI rather than rely solely on glasses to fix the problem. During the camp Leanne went without spectacles as she practiced all the basic games for hyperopia. She filled her bedroom design with vision games.

Q. Teachers, what vision games are important for Leanne?

A. She needs Cross-Crawl and movement for hyperopia, Painting White for reading, and the Bug and Bead game.

Q. Leanne, what do you like?

A. I like Sunning. I like birds and stars.

Six weeks after the Playcamp I received the original optometric report. The diagnosis was accommodative insufficiency. The recommended treatment was near (magnifying) spectacles of +0.75 for both eyes, as a training device. Second, the optometrist wanted Leanne to take a course of in-office exercises with prisms. I explained to Yvonne that when Leanne looked alternately at far and close objects her ciliary muscles and hence the lenses inside her eyes were not responding adequately. That's the accommodation aspect of her case. I suggested that Leanne, and her mother (who was feeling her own vision deteriorate from taking an advanced nursing course), do the Bug and Bead game at least twice a week. This would give Leanne some control over her own "exercise" program and flex both her accommodation and fusion.

Leanne and her Natural Vision Improvement teacher Lynne Sheppard

Leanne's room

Yvonne's follow-up report was that Leanne was doing Bird Swings and Palming, and her schoolteacher was letting her Palm in class. "I took her back to the optometrist right after your course and he found her eyes had improved. He asked me what we had been doing."

I interviewed Leanne, who related, "When I first started to forget to wear my glasses, when I put them on again, it goes all blurry." To my question, "What vision games are you doing and when?" Leanne replied, "I'm using Palming a fair bit . . . like my eyes go all tired and they want to rest. It's a bit like when you wake up in the morning. Normally I think about snow. I see a white bunny go by, a house, a white bed, a ball, maybe a white pillow somewhere. Normally I feel pretty good if I do it that much. Then my eyes feel really good."

## Outdoor Play Areas

All children need time outdoors. After sedentary, mental games indoors, send everyone outdoors for raucous romping. At ChildVision Playcamps every child has equal indoor and outdoor time. All the Natural Vision Improvement games in this book can be played outdoors. To add to the challenge we set up obstacle courses for children to run, with and without eye patches. This simple equipment can easily be set up at home or school. Leave the equipment standing so children can hone their motor and vision skills when no one is watching.

Make crawling spaces from chairs and tables. Secure old tires set in wooden brackets to crawl through. Set up traffic cones for running figure

Margo and Daniel run the snake.

eights and snake patterns. We made traffic cones out of pink and yellow plastic flower pots. The pots can be tacked to a square piece of plywood to keep them stable.

Make a walking board. All children love to walk along cliffs. The safest cliff is a walking board. One sturdy long plank placed on two thick blocks of wood will suffice.

Use garbage bins for "touch goals" and "safe areas."

For more ideas on developing perceptual and motor skills for use at home, consult Jack Capon's book *Perceptual-Motor Lesson Plans*, Levels 1 and 2. If you'd rather have a folkloric, right-brain list of children's games, find *Carmen Out to Play: A Collection of Children's Playground Games*, compiled by Heather Russell. This book includes a number of games children teach one another: Colors Hopscotch, Mother May I?, Five Stones, and Fortune Teller. The rules for these games are never fixed.

Margot walks the plank.

# 20

# The Hazardous Classroom

## History of Western Schooling

Schooling in the United States formed a model for the world. Academic methodology was based on the ideals of Benjamin Rush (1745–1813), a chemist and social reformer and the most famous physician of his time. NVI teacher and sociology professor Raymond Welch made the following comments on Rush's plans for the American schoolchild: "In Rush's mind, schooling in the new Republic should be an advanced form of preventive social therapy. Almost all theorists and social planners of that age, European and American, agreed with Rush that the first concern of public schooling was not the formal subject matter as such, but the character of the young citizen. The moulding of good citizens became and remains the basic goal of the public school."

This presumes the taming of spontaneous urges and the creation of a tractable, conservative, and respectable youngster, a young citizen given to punctuality, discipline, and order.

In Rush's ideal school, children were assigned small, fixed rectangular desks, arranged in rows. The drills for the day were to be strictly governed by allotted time segments and consisted of memorization and recitation. In his essays Rush decreed that future generations were to be fitted into institutions laid down in the present: the masses were to be taught to acquiesce to the plans of the leaders. Schools were to replace the moral and social power of churches in colonial America and Europe.

As democracy spread through Europe and more freedom was given to the common person, a system for controlling that freedom was set in place.

In 1990 the optometrist Raymond Gottlieb, who had improved his own sight with the Bates Method, described myopia in the *Brain-Mind Bulletin* as the "suppression of spontaneous urges."

Before you think I'm putting all the blame for vision problems on the poor old school system, let me firmly state that social structures remain intact only through our acquiescence and cooperation. This gives us as parents the power to change schooling and what happens for our children in classrooms.

# New Hazards for Old

Schools have changed, I am told. They are not as rigid as they used to be. Why, then, are more children developing vision problems as soon as they go to school? On the other hand, books such as *The Learning Revolution* by Gordon Dryden and Jeannette Vos remind us that "the home is the most important educational institution in the land." Fifty percent of a person's ability to learn is developed in the first four years of life and another 30 percent by age eight. Carl Doman's book *Teach Your Baby to Read* has inspired many parents to flash reading cards in the cradle. Myopia at age four, instead of age seven, may be the result.

Children are slaves to the ambitions of parents and governments. The first schools were free. Not free in the sense of paying money but free in the sense that you did not have to go. When schooling became compulsory until age fifteen in many English-speaking countries, some parents revolted; so did some teachers. Homeschooling began, and alternative schools were set up.

Consider the Rudolph Steiner philosophy of child raising. Every child develops in distinct phases. Left-brain scholastics out of phase with natural growth steal life energy from the child. The result is weakness and vulnerability to stress later in life. Steiner-oriented schools provide low-key environments for children to explore at their own pace. Music, art, wooden toys, poetry, and rhymes are the modes through which science and math are explored. A German survey showed that Steiner-school graduates do well at university while maintaining humanitarian inclinations.

My daughter attended three different kinds of schools in her academic training period. The first was based on the values of Wilhelm Reich and of A. S. Neill, founder of the Summerhill School in England. The second, called Westland, was imbued with the notions of John Dewey—the "hands-on" learning man. We then ran out of alternative possibilities, and she entered public school for secondary education.

Cybele shares her experience in alternative and regular schools:

I remember playing a lot at Gateway. We were always doing something, engaging in some sort of exploration. This would be punctuated by a voice calling out that reading was happening, or maths, and everyone would go running; it was where the action was. The learning often took place in a circle on the floor, everyone taking turns. We put on plays from Dr. Seuss and other books. It was fantastic.

Later at Westland the curriculum was more regimented. Each class had a certain theme to explore. Grade threes were Harbour Masters. Grade fours were American Pioneers. Grade fives were Mexicans and Shopkeepers. With each theme we found ourselves pretending to be the characters we were learning about. This was done through crafts, food, clothing, plays, and a final presentation at the end of the semester to our parents. As Shopkeepers in grade five, we all took turns selling paper and other supplies to all the other grades. When I think back on the idea of the six- and seven-year-old class treasurers, lists in hand, going to ten-year-olds to buy tempera paint, I smile.

Year six was my first year at a public school. My first of dreading school, and my first physical fight. Year eight I went to a private college-preparatory school. They provided us with coffee and donuts every morning; well, orange juice and milk too. I later attended a number of different secondary schools, but even the "alternative" ones left me feeling cheated by a lack of joy in learning I had experienced earlier in my education. I didn't find it again at university either.

Cybele, three years old, at Gateway School

## Posture and Seeing

A child's body is pliable and will mold itself to an unsuitable desk. Desks stay rigid like a pair of glasses; young bodies collapse into habitual slumps. Darell Boyd Harmon's classroom study caused school designers to throw out the big tables that children of all sizes had to adapt to. They were replaced by individual chairs because children do not come in the same packaging. Yet posture is still a problem when sitting at a computer, as many adults have learned from the pain between the shoulder blades.

Good posture can be encouraged in several ways. First pay attention to the furniture and lighting situation in the classroom and at home. The second area is energetic and emotional. When a child feels defeated and a failure because she is either zipping ahead of everyone else or lagging behind in the standards set for all the children in the grade, then we get a failure or frustration posture. The central meridian energy flow collapses. The thoughts running through your child's mind when sitting humped over her midline is "I'm a failure." The opposite is "I'm a success."

The command "Sit up straight!" is a shock to the nervous system. More effective is a discussion about the child's attitude toward life. Using Melting Beach Balls to resolve success and failure feelings can restore a child's central meridian flow. Central meridian energy runs from earth to sky, filling both right and left hemispheres of the brain with life energy. You can also use your hand to scoop up earth energy and bring it up the midline of your body to restore joy and confidence. Simply bring your hand from groin to chin three times in a row, imagining your hand is full of flowing vital energy.

The Alexander Technique was devised by F. M. Alexander, an actor from Tasmania. After losing his voice on the Shakespearean stage, Alexander stopped acting and studied his own postural habits. By watching himself in a mirror, he realized that every time he started to speak he raised his head slightly, effectively constricting his vocal cords. Alexander teachers can be found in many countries. Their work releases body energy in relationship to eyes. My first vision student in Los Angeles was Alexander instructor Judith Stransky. I gave her vision lessons and she helped with my posture. It was a mutually beneficial trade. If your child is slumping or her shoulders are rigid and high, Alexander lessons could restore her free and natural stance.

The central meridian

##  Emotional Healing for Going to School

The general word/thought patterns for school are:

> I'm a success.    I'm a failure.

Use the energy Beach Balls. Put the statement "I'm a failure" in your right hand. Give that ball a color and a size and a weight. Repeat the words "I'm a failure" in lots of different ways: sad, angry, don't-care-anyway, or scared, until you can celebrate it and feel the love streaming toward you even when you are a failure. (Sometimes you are.)

When you are satisfied and have broadcast your message of "I'm a failure" over hill and dale, ask what is the opposite of "I'm a failure." You may come up with a different sentence from mine. Maybe you have "I can do anything" or "I'm a genius." Put whatever statement you wish into your left hand. Turn it into a giant energy ball—or a tiny glowing magical gleaming energy ball made of titanium and gold. Announce and explore this thought until you think your two Beach Balls somehow equal each other.

Melt, dissolve, squish the two balls together. Bring your hands to your heart and release the matter. Have a wonderful time learning in your own way, even if you have to go to school. You may come to love school as you expand your capacity to love everything in your life.

Some parents have told me that their child is intensely competitive. Being competitive used to mean desiring success in the world. Times have changed. Stress in the business world results in personalities who make a lot of money and die young of heart attacks. Big business is now looking for teamwork and cooperation rather than "get ahead of the competition" personalities. Human survival now requires practiced and automatic cooperation.

Competitive thought patterns derive from not accepting oneself as a significant being in a supportive universe. A competitive attitude results in a fighting stance, even in the shower. Trapezius and neck flexors never let go. Constant competition reverses the governing meridian. To help your child release a competitive stance and rock-hard shoulders, do Melting Beach Balls with the following thought and word patterns:

I have to compete with others.    I accept myself just as I am.

The governing meridian. Arrows show direction of life energy flow.

# A Great Day for Eyes at School

Could all schools be better for children? Could going to school actually help children develop excellent eyesight instead of poor eyesight? This possibility is a movie in my mind starring Janet Goodrich Method teacher Phil McManus and his daughter Emma:

"Hello, Emma, what did you do at school today?"

"In the morning we went outdoors and Sunned our eyes for a little while. Then we played ball. Catch. At first we were close together, then we got farther and farther apart. Dad, I could catch a ball this tiny all the way from the end of the playing field. Without any glasses. I'll show you. Then we laid down in the grass while Margaret read us a story about an inventor. The guy who made airplanes. Kitty Hawk, that was the place. I remember it because we were Palming while Margaret read and when she said that place I made it into a cat and a bird in my mind.

"Then we went inside. Michael gave us giant pieces of paper. We pasted them to the walls. I made lazy eights all over them to music. I can do hundreds of lazy eights. Look, I'll show you how in the dirt here. Lazy eights make a light go on in your head.

"Tuesday we're going on a boat trip to watch the whales. We have some pictures to identify different seabirds and fish. So we hold the picture in our hands and do Near-Far Swings out to the birds. I'm going to see a dolphin. I can see them already in my head diving around. Sometimes they save people.

"Did you know, Dad, that when people are relaxed they can see better?

"I'll go get some music and show you how to do the Cross-Crawl dance. I do it every time before my math. It helps a lot. Put your right hand like this on your left knee. . . ."

# Children in the Fast Lane

Children either go for technology or reject it completely. A four-year-old in Singapore who was once bright and rambunctious sits listlessly in a chair after coming home from kindergarten. What doesn't he like about school? Children must learn to use a computer.

In Vancouver I see an eight-year-old child daily glued to the screen, body hunched over his joystick, eyes engrossed in Nintendo. What are parents to do in these cases? The response must be individualized, but it is obvious that in the first child a voice cries out, "I don't want to be required to learn via a flat screen at my age." The second child would probably scream bloody murder if his color monitor were taken away. He says, "This is the best thing in my life."

Restriction, deprivation, caving in to cultural values: none of these policies "from above" will have a beneficial effect. Parents will need to get more involved in the life of their child, internally and externally. They may need to change their own values. Parents definitely must make their own choices based on awareness of their child's needs, the possibilities available, and what best fosters health and happiness.

Until now, parents have been cooperating in the creation of a myopic culture. There is a fear that their child will not do well in school or not be able to read the blackboard from the back of the room. The phrase is "Keep up!" with others, who are also trapped in the race. This behavior on the part of parents can end up as the "hurry sickness" from which modem suburbanites are suffering. Parents overrule their initial instinctive questioning of putting a child in glasses. Some parents even agree to the prescription of one-fourth of a diopter correction. This is the minimum curve that can be ground into a lens.

# Parents Make It Happen

## Challenges

To summarize, these are the areas that you face as parent or caretaker of a child with a pair of eyes:

- The patronizing attitude of government and doctors
- Your own fear that your child will somehow be crippled or hindered if her vision is not corrected immediately with an optical device
- The pressure of your peers and family members
- The fear of your child's "falling behind" in school
- Your own lack of confidence
- Your child's current dependence on glasses, either physical or emotional
- Fear that your child may not take to the vision games, either because she is not inspired or (more often) because of negative associations with "eye doctor stuff"

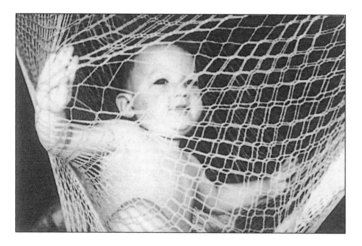

Protecting children from the fast lane trap is a challenge.

The only way to escape being controlled by this list is to realize that your love for children is all-powerful. Within you is still your initial gift of life energy. Bring out your inner child as a healing companion to your offspring. Give the child within yourself, and the child under your care, a chance to escape the trap!

# Assets and Support

Always hold the following in your sights:

- You are your own authority.
- Fear projects illusions into the future; fear is not reality.
- There is a universal healing force operative in your child.
- Confidence comes from experience. You don't have to know everything right now. Start with a baby step.
- Children will prefer not to use glasses once emotional ties and threats are removed.
- Vision games shared with enthusiasm are irresistible and effective.
- You will find professionals, friends, and family members who will be supportive.

When you are down and it looks like nothing is working right, sing the songs on page 228. "The Chinese Meridian Song" combines self-encouragement, transmuting thought patterns, and reviving energy flow through your whole body. Each statement in this song has an effect on the meridian noted and it's corresponding organ, body part, or function.

The chant "Let This Child See" invokes the divine power of grace and unconditional love.

In the eyes of the child, you see the origins of life. All superficial layers of conditioning are swept away in moments of joy. This is perfect sight, and it exists in every one of us!

# THE CHINESE MERIDIAN SONG

*Music – Traditional, Words by Janet Goodrich*

It's O.-K. to win or lose, win or lose, win or lose.
(central: brain, eyes)
It's O.-K. to win or lose, morn-ing, noon and night-time.

I accept me as I am, as I am, as I am... (governing: spine, ears)
It's O.K. to change and grow, change and grow, change and grow... (liver: change)
All my needs are satisfied, satisfied, satisfied... (stomach: digestion)
It's O.K. to look at me... (lung: shame, pride)
It's O.K. to see so far... (kidney: fear of life, love of life)
It's O.K. to see up close... (small intestine: assimilation, learning)
It's O.K. to fuse my eyes. (gall bladder: making choices)
I love seeing, yes I do... (heart: self-love)

# LET THIS CHILD SEE

*Words and Melody by Janet Goodrich*

Let_____ this child see,
Let_____ this child see.    see.

# Glossary

ACCOMMODATION The ability of the visual system to see clearly both distant and close (*see also* CILIARY MUSCLE).

AMBLYOPIA (LAZY EYE) Reduced vision uncorrectable by glasses. It occurs when the brain "switches off" the messages coming from a particular eye. This eye sometimes turns to one side or the other.

ARMORING A word coined by Wilhelm Reich to describe chronic tightness of body muscles resulting from repression of emotional feelings. Armoring may manifest itself in eye muscles as well as in other parts of the body.

ASTIGMATISM Blurring of lines at a particular angle, caused by warping across the cornea and sometimes the lens of the eye. Astigmatism comes and goes and is affected by stress, eyestrain, posture, and emotional factors.

AUTONOMIC NERVOUS SYSTEM The part of our nervous system that functions automatically and is in charge of maintaining a stable internal environment.

BATES METHOD Techniques for relaxing and mobilizing the whole visual system devised by American ophthalmologist William H. Bates. This method emphasized the connection between the body and mind and gave individuals a way to improve their sight without depending on glasses.

BEHAVIORAL OPTOMETRY A specialized branch of optometry that recognizes the influence of environment, posture, and general health on eyesight. The treatment is a combination of training lenses and eye exercises.

BILIRUBIN The red/yellow pigment found in bile, blood, and urine.

CATARACT A pathological eye disease in which the lens of the eye is clouded.

CHI The Chinese term for universal life energy.

CHIROPRACTIC A system of healing based upon the theory that disease results from a lack of normal nerve function. Treatment consists of manipulation and specific adjustments of body structures, especially the spinal column.

CILIARY MUSCLE The muscle that encircles the lens of the eye. It contracts and releases, changing the shape of the lens, thus producing accommodation.

CONCAVE LENS A lens that curves inward, used to compensate for myopia. This lens makes things look smaller.

CONE CELLS Specialized nerve cells on the retina that produce color and detail vision.

CONVEX LENS A lens that curves outward, used to compensate for hyperopia. This lens magnifies.

CORNEA The transparent front of the eye that covers the iris and pupil.

CORPUS CALLOSUM An area of the brain composed of neural fibers that interconnect the hemispheres. This "bridge" between the hemispheres allows them to share memory and learning and to work together.

CROSS-CRAWL A remedial self-help action that reaffirms the bilateral patterning laid down during the crawling stage of infancy. This action combines physical movements requiring simultaneous input from both the left and right hemispheres of the brain. Through this movement both sides are stimulated, "switched on," and brought to work together.

DIOPTER The measurement unit used for describing refractive error on prescriptions. One diopter is the refractive power of a lens needed to focus a point of light at a distance of one meter (about one yard).

DIVERGENCE Moving away from a central point or line. A term used to describe eyes that turn outward. (*See also* STRABISMUS.)

DNA (DIOXYRIBONUCLEIC ACID) An acid found in cells that assists in the transfer of genetic information.

DOMINANT Commanding or controlling. This term is used to describe the sides of the brain and body that are used first; that is, individuals are either right- or left-brain dominant, dictating their particular tendencies even when they are using both sides (*see* RIGHT BRAIN and LEFT BRAIN). A right-handed individual can be described as "right-hand dominant."

DYSLEXIA A state in which an individual has "switched off" part of his or her abilities, usually owing to stress or trying too hard. This may result in slow reading, reversal of letters when writing, or disruption of personal expressiveness.

EMMETROPIA Normal refractive condition of the eye.

ENZYMES Chemicals created by living cells that catalyze processes in the body. The most well-known enzymes are those used by the body for digesting foods. Digestive enzymes are essential for the breaking down of foods into their nutrient components for use by the body.

ESOPHORIA The tendency of eyes to deviate (turn) inward (toward the nose).

ESOTROPIC This describes an eye that turns inward (cross-eyed; *see* PHORIA).

EXOPHORIA The tendency of eyes to deviate outward (away from the nose).

EXOTROPIC This describes an eye that turns outward (wall-eyed; *see* PHORIA).

FAVORING THE PHORIA Referred to when playing vision games. The turning eye (*see* PHORIA) is stimulated to resume a normal line of vision, opposite the direction that the eye is turning.

FOVEA CENTRALIS The point of keenest vision in the eye, located inside the macula lutea. In this area a very large number of cone cells are massed tightly together. When light enters the lens and is cast directly on the fovea centralis, sharp, detailed images will result.

FOVEAL VISION Sharp, clear vision achieved by the fovea centralis. Also called "nuclear" or "central" vision (*see* NUCLEAR VISION).

FUSION The brain and mind's ability to create one image from the messages coming from both eyes.

FUSIONAL RESERVE A reserve of strength and energy in the visual system that allows clear vision and fusion to take place through periods of strain. This reserve lasts for a certain period and can be "recharged" but will not be maintained through long periods of constant stress.

GATE The appearance of two fingers that arises when one finger is held up close in front of the eyes and the attention is in the distance. This image shows that fusion is happening in the visual system.

GLAUCOMA A pathological eye disease characterized by abnormal fluid pressure within the eyeball.

GREAT WHITE GLOW The white aura seen around letters and words when viewing black print on white paper with a relaxed mind.

HEMISPHERE The right or left half of the brain.

HOLISTIC The person is regarded as a whole being made up of physical, emotional, mental, and spiritual components. In healing, the opposite of regarding symptoms in isolation.

HOMOLATERAL Using only one side of the brain or body. This can result in an inability to perform creatively, express spontaneously, and maintain health. Homolateral movement is the opposite of the Cross-Crawl.

HYPEROPIA (FARSIGHTEDNESS) A state in which images of close objects fall behind the retina rather than on it, resulting in visual blur. The physical aspect is an abnormally short eyeball. The emotional aspect is discomfort with closeness, intimacy, details. Usually compensated for by prescription of magnifying, or plus, lenses.

INTEGRATION The merging and blending of abilities and characteristics. The act of unifying rather than isolating. Denotes a state of high human ability.

JAUNDICE A yellowish discoloration of the skin, mucous membranes, and body fluids caused by an excess of bilirubin. Not uncommon in newborns, the most widely known remedy is placing the infant in direct sunlight for short periods.

LEFT BRAIN The left hemisphere of the brain; its abilities and actions. These include counting, analyzing, verbalizing, reasoning, and trying.

LENS The transparent, layered, curved structure that sits between the pupil and vitreous humor. The lens gently bends entering light and helps bring it to a point on the retina.

LIFE ENERGY The universal creative force that brings all beings into life and restores them to a state of balance and health when they go off track.

LYMPHATIC BOUNCING Small gentle jumps by an individual on a minitrampoline that create sufficient muscular movement and gravitational pull to move lymph fluid through the body.

LYMPHATIC SYSTEM A major component of our immune system, the lymphatic system is composed of a clearish fluid that carries proteins, hormones, and fats to all body cells. It carries toxins away from cells, produces antibodies, and manufactures one-fourth of our white blood cells. It is unlike the vascular system of blood transport in the body, which is moved by the action of the heart pumping the blood. Instead, lymph fluid is pumped through the body by the movement of muscles.

MACULA LUTEA A small area on the retina in a direct line back from the lens of the eye. It has a higher concentration of the cone receptor cells than the rest of the retina.

MELANIN A pigment in human skin. It helps to protect the skin from overexposure to sunlight.

MELATONIN A hormone that is stimulated by light. Melatonin affects the brain as well as other glands, such as the adrenals, pituitary, testes, and ovaries. It is also involved in regulating sleeping cycles. It may function as a stress hormone and can affect sexual development.

MINITRAMPOLINE A small trampoline often used indoors. These are available from a numbers of manufacturers and vary in price according to the quality. They usually measure approximately one meter (one yard) across.

MYOPIA (NEARSIGHTEDNESS) A state of the visual system in which images of distant objects fall in front of rather than on the retina, resulting in blur. Physically, the eyeball is too long. Emotionally, myopes usually have difficulty wanting to see or open up to the larger world. Usually compensated for by prescription of contractive, or minus, lenses.

NATURAL VISION IMPROVEMENT (NVI)—THE JANET GOODRICH METHOD A method of improving eyesight by holistic means, without the use of optical devices. Comprising the Bates Method creatively merged with principles of brain function, psychology, and general health, NVI combines working with the physical state of the visual system, the emotional and mental state of the individual, and lifestyle habits.

NEUROLYMPHATIC The lymphatic system is part of the immune system of the body. Neurolymphatic reflexes and points are those relating to the interaction between the nervous and lymphatic systems.

NEUROVASCULAR REFLEXES/POINTS Reflexes involving both nervous and vascular structures (nerves and blood vessels). Points located mainly on the head that stimulate and regulate parts of the nervous and vascular systems.

NUCLEAR VISION A term coined by Janet Goodrich to describe centralized, crystal-clear foveal vision. Mentally the object regarded is seen more clearly than anything surrounding it. Physically the light from the object regarded falls into the fovea centralis (see FOVEAL VISION).

OBLIGATION (as used in this book) The requirement to perform to a certain standard. In the case of eye tests, this "obligation to perform" in itself creates a stressful situation that can result in visual blur.

OCULAR ANESTHESIA Anesthesia used on the eye so that surgery can be performed.

OPHTHALMOLOGIST A medical doctor specializing in examining eyes and prescribing glasses and diagnosing and treating eye diseases. Performs optional surgeries for strabismus and myopia.

OPTIC CHIASM The intersection of the optic nerves from the two eyes. At this point in the brain the optic nerve fibers divide, half from each eye crossing over to join half from the other eye.

OPTOMETRIST Examines eyes and prescribes glasses. Diagnoses but usually refers eye diseases. (See also BEHAVIORAL OPTOMETRY.)

ORTHOPTICS A medically accepted method of exercising eye muscles to correct crossed eyes and muscular weakness. Commonly used for a short period after surgery.

OSTEOPATH A practitioner of osteopathy.

OSTEOPATHY A system of medical treatment based on the theory that diseases are chiefly due to the loss of structural integrity in the tissues of the body. Treatment consists of body manipulation (adjustments), surgery, drugs, and diet.

PALMING Gently placing the cupped palms of the hands over closed eyes to relax by visualizing pleasant images.

PATCHING Covering one eye with an obscuring material to encourage the uncovered eye to wake up, perceive, and strengthen.

PHORIA The tendency of lines of vision to deviate from the normal. (See also ESOPHORIA, EXOPHORIA, FAVORING THE PHORIA.)

PITUITARY GLAND The body's "concertmaster," which secretes hormones that regulate the endocrine system.

PTERYGIUM A fleshy mass of conjunctiva that usually occurs at the inner side of the eyeball, covering part of the cornea. Pterygiums can cause a disturbance of vision by growing across the pupil.

REFLEX A physical movement or internal change performed automatically and without conscious volition. Nerve impulses sent from various parts of the body are received by the brain, which sends back an instant and automatic response. There are several different kinds of reflexes in the human body. The important ones for healing are messages passed between muscular, organ, and nerve systems.

REFLEX POINT A small area in a specific location on the body. When stimulated, these points send information and energy to the relevant organ, muscles, or nerve system, which helps in activating and regulating their function.

REFRACTIVE ERROR A deviation in the eye's ability to bend incoming light to create a clear image. Variations are labeled as hyperopia, myopia, presbyopia ("old-age sight"), and astigmatism.

REICHIAN THERAPY A method of changing human unhappiness by freeing breathing patterns and increasing the flow of biological energy through the body. Reichian principles and practices incorporate natural childbirth, self-regulation and self-responsibility, positive sexual and emotional expression, and human autonomy.

REM (RAPID EYE MOVEMENT) Prior to periods of deep sleep, an individual's eyes make many rapid small movements behind closed lids.

RETINA The responsive layer of specialized nerve cells at the back of the eye that change light into electrical impulses.

RETINOSCOPE An optical instrument that casts a beam of light into the eye, revealing whether it is in a state of refractive error.

RETINOSCOPY Objective examination of the refractive powers of the eye by observation with a retinoscope.

RIGHT BRAIN The right hemisphere of the brain; its abilities and actions. These include rhythmic movement through space, imaging, musicality, and supplying balanced energy to all body muscles.

ROD CELLS Nerve cells in the retina that register light and dark. They are stimulated in dim light and do not register color.

SACCADES Quick, small movements that enable the eyes to pick up details and to move from one object of interest to another.

SEASONAL AFFECTIVE DISORDER (SAD) An affliction suffered by people who live in areas of long winters, with short daylight periods. A lack of sufficient light (sunlight) causes depression and malaise.

SELF-REGULATION A principle used in child-centered schooling and nurturing. Children determine their own activities and schedules. Best understood as meaning freedom, not license.

SQUINT (see STRABISMUS)

STRABISMUS Turning of an eye so that both eyes are unable to look at the same point simultaneously.

SUNNING Relaxing for short periods in the sunlight with eyes closed. Sunning allows body and eyes to absorb the small amount of UV light essential to human health.

SWING Moving attention and body to relax and to activate rapid saccadic movement in the eyes.

TOUCH FOR HEALTH A system for laypeople to correct and restore body energy using muscle testing. Pressure points on the body are activated to improve posture and relieve headaches, indigestion, and other ailments before the underlying imbalances result in disease.

TRANSITION GLASSES (T-GLASSES) Under-corrected glasses worn by Natural Vision Improvement students that give eyes room for change and allow the student to see adequately when necessary.

TROMBONING Covering one eye with the palm and moving an object near and far to strengthen and flex the components of accommodation.

ULTRAVIOLET (UV) LIGHT That part of the sun's rays with slightly greater frequency than violet. It is also emitted by artificial lamps that are used for healing, growing plants, and forming vitamins.

Ultraviolet is said to be necessary for human health, as it stimulates the pituitary gland.

UV LIGHT *See* ULTRAVIOLET LIGHT.

VISUAL CORTEX A part of the cerebral cortex in the brain, primarily responsible for interpreting visual impulses from the eyes. Also called the visual brain.

# References

## Chapter 1

Bates, W. H. *The Bates Method for Better Eyesight without Glasses.* Jove Publications, 1978.

Corbett, Margaret. *Help Yourself to Better Sight.* New York: Prentice Hall, 1949.

Duke-Elder, Sir Stewart. *The Practice of Refraction*, 7th ed. London: J & A Churchill, 1963.

Gesell, Arnold, Frances Ilg, and Glenna Bullis. *Vision: Its Development in Infant and Child.* New York: Paul B. Hoeber, 1949.

Hammel, Faye. "The Myopia Epidemic," *New York Sunday News* magazine, May 18, 1980.

Harmon, Darell Boyd. *The Co-ordinated Classroom.* Booklet, 1951.

Huxley, Aldous. *The Art of Seeing, An Adventure in Re-education.* New York: Harper & Brothers, 1942.

Lierman, Emily. *Stories from the Clinic.* New York: Central Fixation, 1926.

[...]lph Mae, and the editors [...]ght and Vision. New York:

[...] M.D., ed. *Manual of [...]rapy*, 3d ed. Boston: [...]91.

[...]and Orgonomy. New York:

Reich, Wilhelm. *Selected Writings: An Introduction to Orgonomy.* Noonday Press, 1973.

———. *The Function of the Orgasm.* London: Souvenir Press.

Thie, John F. *Touch for Health.* Santa Monica, Calif.: DeVorss & Co., 1979.

Wertenbaker, Lael. *The Eye: Window to the World.* Torstar Books: 1984.

Yarbus, Alfred L. *Eye Movements and Vision.* New York: Plenum Press, 1967.

*Myopie Kann Nicht Trainiert Werden.* DVA, 1989.

## Chapter 2

Committee on Vision, National Research Council. *Myopia: Prevalence and Progression.* Washington, D.C.: National Academy Press, 1989.

Duke-Elder. *The Practice of Refraction.*

Goodrich, J. "Reichian Therapy: The Visual Block." Unpublished dissertation, Antioch University Without Walls, 1976.

Kelley, Charles R. "Psychological Factors in Myopia," *Journal of the American Optometric Association* 33, no. 6 (1967): 833–37.

LaSalle, Coralee. "Psychological Changes in Bates Method Students." Unpublished dissertation, University of California–Los Angeles, 1975.

Proc, K. Van Alphen. "A Comparative Psychological Investigation in Myopes and Emmetropes," *Nederl. Akad. Wet.* 55, no. 5 (1951): 689–96.

Sekuler, Robert and Patrick Mulvanny. "20/20 Is Not Enough," *American Health,* November/December 1982.

Subcommittee on Vision and Its Disorders. *Emmetropia and Ametropia, in Refractive Anomalies,* NINDS Monograph 5. Bethesda, Md.: U.S. National Advisory Neurological Diseases and Blinding Council, 1967.

Young, F. A., G. A. Leary, W. R. Baldwin, and D. C. West. "The Transmission of Refractive Errors within Eskimo Families," *American Journal of Optometry* 46 (1969): 676–85.

## Chapter 3

Flax, Nathan, and Robert Duckman. "Orthoptic Treatment of Strabismus," *Journal of the American Optometric Association* 49, no. 12, 1978.

Gillett, Geoff. Medicare Program Branch, Health Insurance Commission, Tuggeranong, Australian Capital Territory, Australia.

Kavner, Richard S. *Your Child's Vision: A Parent's Guide to Seeing, Growing, and Developing.* New York: Simon and Schuster, 1985.

Letter, House of Representatives Committee on Post Office and Civil Service, May 11, 1982, to Clinton R. Miller, then Executive Director, National Health Federation, Monrovia, Calif.

Liberman, Jacob. *Take Off Your Glasses and See.* New York: Crown Books, 1995.

Orfield, Antonia. "Seeing Space: Undergoing Brain Re-programming to Reduce Myopia," *Journal of Behavioral Optometry* 5, 1994.

Thompson, Graeme. Personal communication.

## Chapter 5

Dawson, Cameron. Personal communication, June 2, 1995.

*Geo Wissen* magazine (Germany), no. 2, September 1993.

Gesell, Ilg, and Bullis. *Vision.*

Magoun, Harold I., ed. *Osteopathy in the Cranial Field,* 2nd ed. Kirksville, Mo.: Journal Printing Company, 1966.

Rapoport, Carla. "Charles Handy Sees the Future," *Time* magazine, February 13, 1995.

Schell, Robert E., and Elizabeth Hall. *Developmental Psychology Today,* 4th ed. New York: Random House, 1983.

Silverstein, Samuel. *Child Spirit.* Santa Fe, N.M.: Bear & Co., 1991.

## Chapter 6

Leboyer, Frederick. *Loving Hands.* London: Collins, 1977.

Walther, David S. "Basic Procedures and Muscle Testing Systems," *Applied Kinesiology* 1, 1981.

## Chapter 7

*Consumers Digest,* "Beware the Baby Walker." January/February 1993.

Dennison, Paul. *Switching On: A Guide to Edu-Kinesthetics.* Glendale, Calif.: Edu-Kinesthetics, 1981.

Diamond, M. C., A. B. Scheibel, and L. M. Elson. *The Human Brain Coloring Book.* New York: Harper & Row, 1985.

Fincher, Jack. *The Brain: Mystery of Matter and Mind.* Washington, D.C.: U.S. News Books, 1981.

Schell and Hall, *Developmental Psychology Today.*

## Chapter 8

Bruna, Dick. *The Fish.* Chicago: Follett Publishing, 1963.

Sea, Jan Fisher. *No Bored Babies: A Guide to Making Developmental Toys for Babies Birth to Age Two.* Seattle, Wash.: Bear Creek Publications, 1990.

Stern, John A. *The Sciences.* New York: New York Academy of Sciences, 1988.

Yarbus. *Eye Movements and Vision.*

## Chapter 9

Hollwich, F. *The Influence of Ocular Light Perception on Metabolism in Man and in Animal*. New York: Springer-Verlag, 1979.

Kime, Zane R. *Sunlight Can Save Your Life*. Penryn, Calif.: World Health Publications, 1980.

Liberman, Jacob. *Light Medicine of the Future*. Santa Fe, N.M.: Bear & Company, 1991.

Ott, John N. "Artificial Light: Plain Common Sense vs. Scientific Theoretical Irrationality," *International Journal of Biosocial Research* 7, 1985.

———. *Health and Light*. Arid Press, 1976.

Samuels, Mike, and Nancy Samuels. *The Well Pregnancy Book*. New York: Summit Books, 1986.

Todd, Gary Price. *Nutrition, Health, and Disease*. Whitford Press, 1985.

## Chapter 10

Farah, Martha J. "Is Visual Imagery Really Visual? Overlooked Evidence from Neuro-Psychiatry," *Psychological Review* 95 (1988): 307–17.

Mueller, Else. *Traeumen auf der Mondschaukel Koesel*. 1993.

## Chapter 11

Busacca, Richard. "The Individual in Society and Culture." San Francisco State University.

Krishnamurti, J. *Krishnamurti to Himself*. London: Victor Gollancz, 1987.

## Chapter 12

Yarbus. *Eye Movements and Vision*.

## Chapter 13

*Consumer Reports Harvard Health Letter*. "Goodbye Glasses?," January 1988.

Gesell, Ilg, and Bullis. *Vision*.

## Chapter 15

Duke-Elder. *The Practice of Refraction*.

## Chapter 16

Dawson, Cameron. Personal communication, June 2, 1995.

Duke-Elder. *The Practice of Refraction*.

Goodrich, Janet. *Natural Vision Improvement*. Melbourne, Australia: Viking Penguin, 1990.

Jacob, Stanley W., and Clarice Ashworth Francone. *Structure and Function in Man*, 3rd ed. Philadelphia: W. B. Saunders, 1974.

Kavner. *Your Child's Vision*.

Samuels, Mike, and Nancy Samuels. *The Well Baby Book*. New York: Summit Books, 1991.

## Chapter 17

Jacob and Francone. *Structure and Function*.

## Chapter 18

Cutter, Karin. "Milk: Is It Really Good for You?," *Well Being Journal*, Sydney, September 1995.

Dufty, William. *Sugar Blues*. New York: Chilton, 1975.

*Health Discoveries Newsletter*. Lafayette Institute for Basic Research, Charlottesville, Va.

## Chapter 20

Neill, A. S. *Summerhill: A Radical Approach to Child Rearing*. New York: Hart Publishing, 1960.

Welch, Raymond. *Making a Spectacle World*. Unpublished essay written during training as an NVI teacher in Los Angeles, 1981.

# Recommended Reading

## Child Development

Crockford, Patricia. *Games for Growing Babies.* Australia: Bridgewater Books, 1989.

———. *Games for Growing Toddlers.* Australia: Bridgewater Books, 1989.

———. *Games for Growing Two-Year-Olds.* Australia: Bridgewater Books, 1989.

Fisher Sea, Jan. *No Bored Babies: A Guide to Making Developmental Toys for Babies Birth to Age Two.* Seattle, Wash.: Bear Creek Publications, 1990.

Parker, Allan, and Margaret Cutler-Stuart. *Switch on Your Brain.* Australia: Hale & Iremonger, 1986.

Russell, Heather. *Carmen Out to Play!* Oxford University Press, 1989.

Silverstein, Samuel. *Child Spirit: Children's Experience with God in School.* Santa Fe, N.M.: Bear & Company, 1991.

## Nutrition and Recipe Books

Kenton, Leslie, and Susannah Kenton. *Raw Energy Recipes.* London: Century Publishing, 1985.

O'Dea, Jenny. *Healthy Food Your Kids Will Love!* Australia: Currey O'Neil Ross, 1985.

Price Todd, Gary. *Acquiring Optimal Health.* Norfolk, Va.: Hampton Roads Publishing, 1994.

Stanton, Rosemary. *Healthy Cooking.* Murdoch Books, 1993.

Stephens, Helen. *The Australian Family Vegetarian Cookbook.* South Melbourne, Vic.: Hyland House Publishing, 1994.

## Picture Books for Children

### Level 1

Bruna, Dick. *The Fish.* Chicago: Follett Publishing, 1963.

———. *Little Bird Tweet.* Chicago: Follett Publishing, 1963.

Pragoff, Fiona. *Baby Says.* HarperCollins, 1994.

### Level 2

Campbell, Rod. *Dear Zoo.* Picture Puffins, 1984.

Hutchins, Pat. *Rosie's Walk.* Picture Puffins, 1970.

### Level 3

Ahlberg, Janet, and Allan Ahlberg. *Each Peach Pear Plum.* Picture Puffins, 1989.

Berrett, Rebecca. *The Junk Drawer.* MacMillan Company of Australia, 1988.

Carle, Eric. *The Bad-Tempered Ladybird.* Picture Puffins, 1982.

Hetherington, Norman, and Margaret Hetherington. *Mr. Squiggle and the Preposterous Purple Crocodile.* Australia: ABC Enterprises, 1993.

Johnson, Crockett. *Harold and the Purple Crayon.* New York: HarperCollins, 1983.

LeSieg, Theo. *Wacky Wednesday.* New York: Random House, 1974.

Wick, Walter, and Jean Marzollo. *I Spy Fantasy: A Book of Picture Riddles.* New York: Scholastic, 1994.

## Level 4

Handford, Martin. *Where's Wally?*, vol. 3, *The Fantastic Journey*. Australia: Century Hutchinson, 1990.

Heimann, Roif. *For Eagle Eyes Only*. Australia: Periscope Press, 1993.

———. *Ultimaze Book*. Australia: Periscope Press, 1993.

Lester, Alison. *Imagine*. Australia: Allen and Unwin, 1992.

———. *The Journey Home*. Oxford University Press, 1990.

Pirani, Felix. *Abigail Goes Visiting*. London: Diamond Books, 1994.

Tallarico, Anthony. *Where's Wendy?* Chicago: Kidsbooks, 1991.

## Level 5

Base, Graeme. *Animalia*. Puffin Books, 1990.

N. E. Thing Enterprises. *The Magic Eye*. Viking, 1993.

de Rico, Ui. *The Rainbow Goblins*. New York: Thames & Hudson, 1978.

Tonkin, Rachel. *Willy and the Ogre*. Australia: Hodder & Stoughton, 1991.

Whatley, Bruce, and Rosie Smith. *Whatley's Quest*. Angus & Robertson, 1994.

## Vision Improvement

Goodrich, Janet. *Natural Vision Improvement* (available at all major bookshops or the NVI head office). Berkeley, Calif.: Celestial Arts, 1986.

Liberman, Jacob. *Take Off Your Glasses and See*. New York: Crown Publishers, 1995.

## Light

Kime, Zane. *Sunlight Can Save Your Life*. Penry, Calif.: World Health Publications.

Liberman, Jacob. *Light: Medicine of the Future*. Rochester, Vermont: Bear & Company, 1991.

## Education

Greenberg, Daniel. *Free At the Last: Sudbury Valley School*. Framingham, Mass.: Sudbury Valley School Press, 1995.

Neill, A. S. *Freedom, Not License!* New York: Hart Publishing, 1966.

———. *Summerhill: A Radical Approach to Child Rearing*. New York: Hart, 1960.

# Resources

## Natural Vision Improvement

For information about locating or training to be an NVI instructor, contact:

Natural Vision Improvement
12 Crystal Waters Village
Maleny, QLD 4552 Australia
Phone: +61 (7) 5494 4888
e-mail: good4nvi@ozemail.com.au
www.naturalvisionimprovement.net.au

Specialized products available from the center:

Natural Vision Improvement Cassettes/CD's talk you through eleven vision games and color visualization activities. For adults and older children, includes eye charts and booklet.
EyeSongs audio cassettes
Eagle Eye poster, trampolines, pinholes, instructional materials

## Movement Education

To purchase books by Jack Capon and for a free catalog of guidebooks for movement education and perceptual-motor development, contact:

Front Row Experience
540 Discovery Bay Boulevard
Byron, CA 94514-9454

Children's motor development classes:

Toddler Kindy Gymbaroo
Parent/Child Education Centres
142 Cotham Rd.
Kew, VIC 3101 Australia
Phone: 800 559 426

## Eye Professionals

Australasian College of Behavioral Optometrists
Bookshop and referrals:
Roberts Alexander and Associates
Strathpine, QLD Australia
Phone: (07) 3205 1593

Baltimore Academy for Behavioral Optometry
110 Old Padonia Road, Suite 300
Cockeysville, MD 21030
Phone: (800) 447-0370
www.babousa.org

Cameron Dawson Technologies for the Dawson Programme
249 Auburn Rd.
Hawthorne, VIC 3122 Australia
Phone: (800) 648 668

Holistic Optometry Association
Jenny Livanos
Phone: (02) 8765 96001

Optometric Extension Program Foundation
1921 E. Carnegie Ave., Suite 3-L
Santa Ana, CA 92705
Phone: (949) 250-8070
e-mail: oep@oep.org
www.oep.org

Pacific University College of Optometry
2043 College Way
Forest Grove, OR 97116
Phone: (800) 933-9308

## Body Workers

American Society for the Alexander Technique
P.O. Box 60008
Florence, MA 01062
Phone: (800) 473-0620
www.alexandertech.org
e-mail: alexandertech@earthlink.net

Australian Society of Teachers of the Alexander
Technique
16 Princes Street
Kew, VIC 3101 Australia
Phone: (800) 339 571

Consult your local phone book for addresses of
osteopathic and chiropractic associations.

## Touch for Health and Educational Kinesiology

Touch for Health Education:
www.touch4health.com

American Academy of Kinesiology and Physical
Education
Human Kinetics
P.O. Box 5076
Champaign, IL 61820
www.aakpe.org

Australian Kinesiology Association
P.0. Box 233
Kerrimuir, VIC 3129
Phone: 0500 503 355

Australian TFH Association
P.O. Box 5088
Frankston South, VIC 3199
Phone: 0500 888 119
www.touch4health.org.au

The British Kinesiology Federation
30 Dudley Road
West Sussex P021 1ER, England
Phone: 243-841-689

North American TFH Association
6955 Fernhill Drive
Malibu, CA 90265
Phone: (310) 457-8342

TFH Association of Canada
Box 74508
Kitsailano Postal Unit
Vancouver BC V6K 4P4
Phone: 604-978-6292

TFH Association of NZ
33 Gilshennan Valley
Red Beach, New Zealand
Phone: (09) 426-7695

## Information on Nutrition and Eye Pathologies

Dr. Gary Price Todd
Bio-Zoe Inc.
P.0. Box 49
Waynesville NC 28786
Phone: (704) 452-0472
Fax: (704) 456-4471

Dr. Lesley Salov
Vision and Health Center
W3064 Piper Road
Whitewater, WI 53190
Phone: (414) 473-7361

# Index

# Books of Related Interest

**THE POWER BEHIND YOUR EYES**
Improving Your Eyesight with Integrated Vision Therapy
*by Robert-Michael Kaplan, O.D.*

**LIGHT: MEDICINE OF THE FUTURE**
How We Can Use It to Heal Ourselves NOW
*by Jacob Liberman, O.D., Ph.D.*

**VACCINATIONS: A THOUGHTFUL PARENT'S GUIDE**
How to Make Safe, Sensible Decisions about the
Risks, Benefits, and Alternatives
*by Aviva Jill Romm*

**NATURAL HEALTH AFTER BIRTH**
The Complete Guide to Postpartum Wellness
*by Aviva Jill Romm*

**CHILDREN AT PLAY**
Using Waldorf Principles to Foster Childhood Development
*by Heidi Britz-Crecelius*

**THE EDISON GENE**
ADHD and the Gift of the Hunter Child
*by Thom Hartmann*

**THE FAMILY HERBAL**
A Guide to Natural Health Care for Yourself and Your
Children from Europe's Leading Herbalists
*by Barbara & Peter Theiss*

**THE ACID–ALKALINE DIET FOR OPTIMUM HEALTH**
Restore Your Health by Creating Balance in Your Diet
*by Christopher Vasey, N.D.*

Inner Traditions • Bear & Company
P.O. Box 388
Rochester, VT  05767
1-800-246-8648
www.InnerTraditions.com

Or contact your local bookseller